MRI made easy

Author: Univ.-Prof. Dr. Hans H. Schild
Radiological University Hospital Bonn / Germany

Acknowledgements

I would like to thank the following people, whose cooperation and expertise made this book possible:

for the first edition:
– Mrs. L. Schmidt, and Dr. H. Weinmann from former "Schering AG",
– Mr. D. Wettstein, and Mr. S. Jacob from "Wettstein Fotosatz",
– Mr. R. Carpenter, and Mr. A. Leihberg,
– Prof. Dr. M. Heller, and special thanks to
– Mr. H. H. Vos also from former "Schering AG";

for the updated edition:
– Mr. Dirk Meissner from "himself" for the cartoons,
– Mr. Stephan Huhn from "STEP-ANI-MOTION" for the technical illustrations,
– Mr. Dietmar Suchalla from "Magazine Factory" for design and layout,
– Mrs. Axinja Munkel from "Bayer HealthCare" for coordination,
– Mr. Manfred Gnegel, external proofreader for "Bayer HealthCare";

and last but by far not least:
– Johannes Weid from "Bayer HealthCare" for supporting the project.

In memory of the late Dr. Hanns Weinmann, and the late Bernhard Dreikorn.

Printed in Germany by
H. Heenemann GmbH & Co. KG
© Copyright by Bayer Pharma AG
Berlin 2012
ISBN 978-3-00-038441-7

G.DI.04.2012.0202

Preface

This book is dedicated

– to anyone, who tries to teach medicine
instead of just reporting medical facts (like my anatomy
teacher, Prof. Dr. R. Bock, who was a master of this art);

– and to anyone, whose stumbling feet find the MRI path difficult

(the book was written in the hope rather than the belief
that they may find some help from it).

(modified from Alastair G. Smith, Surgeons Hall, Edinburgh, October 1939)

H. H. Schild

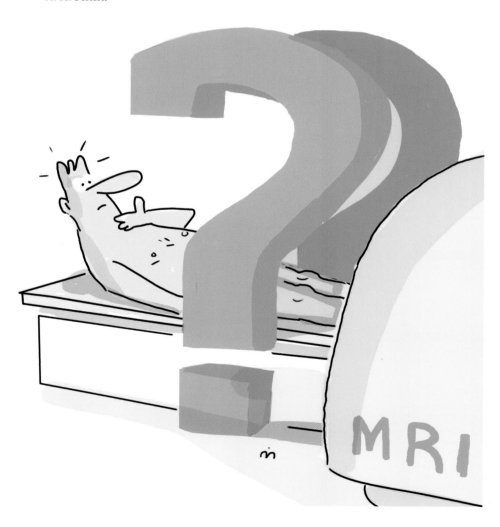

Let us start with a general overview of MRI . . .

The single steps of an MRI examination can be described quite simply:

1. the patient is placed in a magnet,

2. a radio wave is sent in,

3. the radio wave is turned off,

4. the patient emits a signal, which is received and used for

5. reconstruction of the picture.

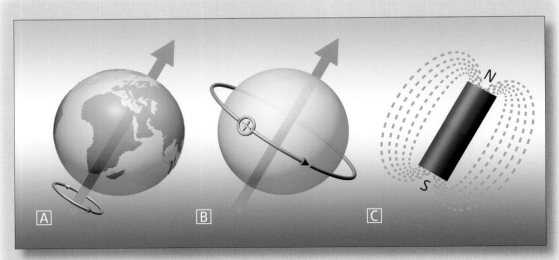

Fig. 1: Protons possess a positive charge. Like the earth, they are constantly turning around an axis and have their own magnetic field.

Let's take a look at these steps in detail

What happens, when we put a patient into the magnet of an MR machine?

To understand this, it is necessary to at least know some very basic physics – even though this may seem to be boring.

As we all know, **atoms** consist of a **nucleus** and a **shell**, which is made up of electrons. In the nucleus – besides other things – there are **protons**, little particles, that have a positive electrical charge (whatever that may actually be). These protons are analogous to little planets. Like the earth, they are constantly turning, or spinning around an axis (figure 1); or – as one says, protons possess a **spin**. The positive electrical charge, being attached to the proton, naturally spins around with it. And what is a moving electrical charge? It is an **electrical current**.

Now, may be you remember from your physics at school that an electrical current induces, causes a **magnetic force**, or **magnetic field**. So, where there is an electrical current, there is also a magnetic field.

Let's review what we have read

A proton has a spin, and thus the electrical charge of the proton also moves. A moving electrical charge is an electrical current, and this is accompanied by a magnetic field. Thus, the proton has its own magnetic field and can be seen as a little **bar magnet** (figure 1C).

What happens to the protons, when we put them into an external magnetic field?

The protons – being little magnets – align themselves in the external magnetic field like a compass needle in the magnetic field of the earth. However, there is an important difference. For the compass needle there is only one way to align itself with the magnetic field, for the protons, however, there are two (figure 2):

The protons may align with their South and North Poles in the direction of the external field, parallel to it. Or they may point in the completely opposite direction, anti-parallel. These types of alignment are on different energy levels. To explain this: a man can align himself parallel to the magnetic field of the earth, i.e. walk on his feet, or he can align himself anti-parallel, in the opposite direction. Both states are on different energy levels, i.e. they need different amounts of energy.

Walking on one's feet is undoubtedly less exhausting, takes less energy than walking on one's hands. (In the figures, this will be illustrated as pointing up or down, see figure 2).

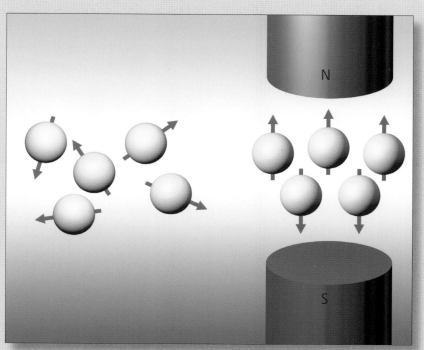

Fig. 2: Normally, protons are aligned in a random fashion. This, however, changes when they are exposed to a strong external magnetic field. Then they are aligned in only two ways, either **parallel** or **anti-parallel** to the external magnetic field.

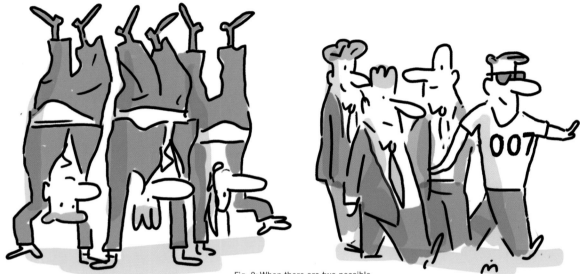

Fig. 3: When there are two possible
states of alignment, the one that
takes less energy, is on a lower
energy level, is preferred.

Naturally, the preferred state of alignment is the one that needs less energy. So more protons are on the lower energy level, parallel to the external magnetic field, walking on their feet, so to speak. A smaller number is on the higher energy level, anti-parallel, "walking on their hands".

The difference in number is, however, very small and depends on the strength of the applied magnetic field. To get a rough idea: for about 10 million protons "walking on their hands", there are about 10,000,007 "walking on their feet". The difference "007" is probably easy to remember, isn't it?

It may be obvious at this point already that for MRI the **mobile protons** are important (which are a subset of all protons that are in the body).

The movement of protons – precession

Let us take a closer look at these protons

We will see that the protons do not just lie there, aligned **parallel** or **anti-parallel** to the magnetic field lines. Instead, they move around in a certain way. The type of movement is called **precession** (figure 4A).

What type of movement is "precession"?

Just imagine a spinning top. When you hit it, it starts to "wobble" or tumble around. It does not, however, fall over. During the precession, the axis of the spinning top circles forming a cone shape (figure 4B). It is hard to draw such a precessing proton, because

this is a very fast movement, as we will see below. For the sake of simplicity, we will just make "freeze frame" pictures, as if we were taking a fast flashlight photograph of the situation at a specific moment in time.

For reasons we will learn later, it is important to know how fast the protons precess. This speed can be measured as precession frequency, that is how many times the protons precess per second. This precession frequency is not constant. It depends upon the strength of the magnetic field (for magnetic field strength, see page 94), in which the protons are placed.

The stronger the magnetic field, the faster the **precession rate** and the higher the **precession frequency**.

This is like a violin string: the stronger the force exerted upon the string, the higher its frequency.

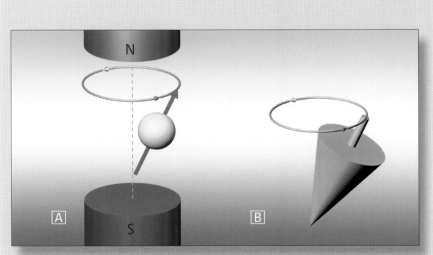

Fig. 4: A spinning top which is hit, performs a wobbling type of motion. Protons in a strong magnetic field also show this type of motion, which is called precession.

It is possible and necessary to precisely calculate this frequency. This is done by using an equation called the **Larmor equation**:

$$\omega_0 = \gamma B_0$$

ω_0 is the **precession frequency** – in Hz or MHz,
B_0 is the strength of the external magnetic field, which is given in **Tesla (T)** (see page 94), and
γ is the so-called **gyro-magnetic ratio**.

The equation states that the precession frequency becomes higher when the magnetic field strength increases. The exact relationship is determined by the gyro-magnetic ratio γ. This gyro-magnetic ratio is different for different materials (e.g. the value for hydrogen protons is 42.5 MHz/T).

It can be compared to an exchange rate, which is different for different currencies.

Time to take a break

However, let us briefly review what we have learned up to now:
● Protons have a positive electrical charge, which is constantly moving, because the protons possess a spin.
● This moving electrical charge is nothing more than an electrical current, and the latter always induces a magnetic field.
● So every proton has its own little magnetic field, and can thus be seen as a little bar magnet.
● When we put a patient in the MR magnet, the protons, being little magnets, align with the external magnetic field. They do this in two ways: parallel

and anti-parallel. The state that needs less energy is preferred, and so there are a few more protons "walking on their feet" than "on their hands" (figure 3).
● The protons precess along the field lines of the magnetic field, just like a spinning top that precesses along the field lines of the magnetic field of earth.
● The precession frequency can be calculated by the Larmor equation, and is higher in stronger magnetic fields. Why is this precession frequency important?

It has something to do with the "resonance" in magnetic resonance imaging. But to understand this will take a few more minutes.

After the break you should go over this last summary again, and then continue ...

Introducing the coordinate system

To make communication (and drawing of illustrations) easier, let us start using a coordinate system like the one used at school (figure 5). As you can see, the z-axis runs in the direction of the magnetic field lines, and thus can represent them. So we can stop drawing the external magnet in all other illustrations.

From here on we will also illustrate the protons as **vectors**, as little arrows.

Maybe you remember: a vector represents a certain force (by its size) that acts in a certain direction (direction of the arrow). The force that is represented by vectors in our illustrations, is the magnetic force.

Fig. 5: Using a coordinate system makes the description of proton motion in the magnetic field easier, and we can also stop drawing the external magnet.

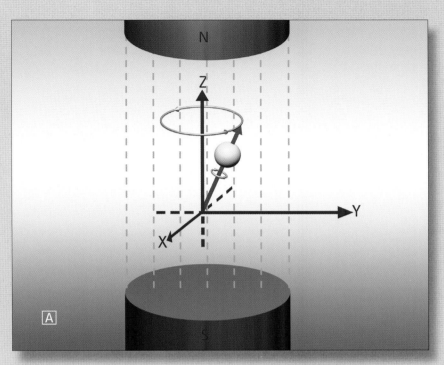

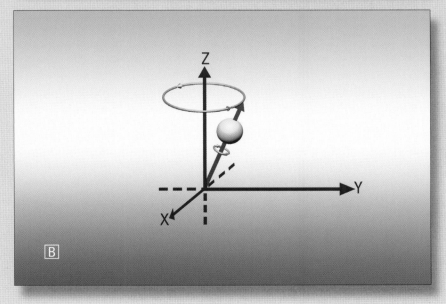

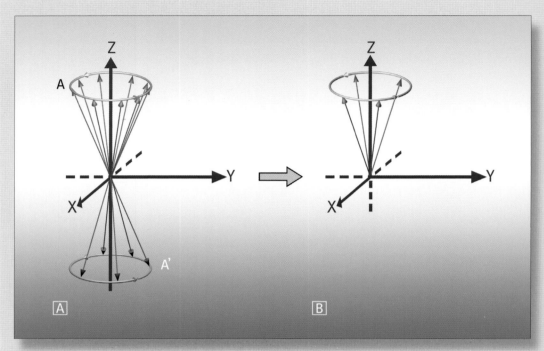

Fig. 6: The five protons, which "point" down, cancel out the magnetic effects of the same number of protons, which "point" up (A). So in effect it is sufficient to look only at the four unopposed protons (B).

Now, let us look at figure 6. Here we have 9 protons pointing up, precessing parallel to the external magnetic field lines, and 5 protons pointing down, precessing anti-parallel to the external magnetic field.

What we see in the figure is just a picture taken at a specific point in time. A picture taken just a little later would show the protons in different positions, because they precess. The precession actually goes very fast, the **precession frequency** for hydrogen protons is somewhere around 42 MHz in a magnetic field strength of 1 Tesla (see page 94); this means that the protons precess around the "ice cream cone" more than 42 million times per second. Now there are millions and millions of pro-

tons in your body precessing this fast. It is easy to imagine that at a certain moment, there may be one proton (A in the illustration) pointing in one direction, and another proton (A') pointing exactly in the opposite direction. The result is very important; the magnetic forces in the opposing directions cancel each other out, like two persons pulling at the opposite ends of a rope. Finally, for every proton pointing down, there is one pointing up, cancelling its magnetic effect. But as we have learned: there are more protons pointing up than down, and the magnetic forces of these protons are not cancelled by others. So we are left – in effect – with some protons (4 in our example) pointing up (figure 6).

Fig. 7: The magnetic force of proton A, illustrated as an arrow, a vector, can be seen as resulting from two components: one pointing up along the z-axis, and one in direction of the y-axis. The component along the y-axis is cancelled out by proton A', the magnetic force of which also has a component along the y-axis, but in the opposite direction. The same holds true for other protons, e.g. B and B', which cancel their respective magnetic vectors along the x-axis. In contrast to the magnetic vectors in the x-y-plane, which cancel each other out, the vectors along the z-axis point in the same direction, and thus add up to a new magnetic sum vector pointing up.

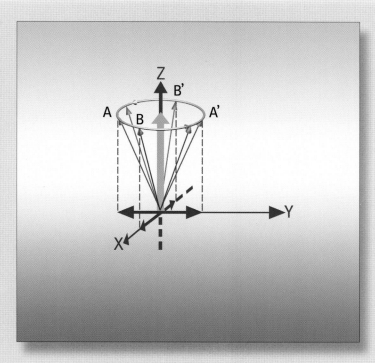

However, not only magnetic forces pointing up and down can cancel or neutralize each other. As the protons that are pointing up, precess, there may be one pointing to the right, while another one is pointing to the left; or for one pointing to the front, there is one pointing backwards, and so on (the corresponding protons in figure 7 are marked A and A', B and B' for example). This means that the opposing magnetic forces of the remaining protons cancel each other out in these directions. This is true for all but one direction, the direction of the z-axis, along the external magnetic field (figure 7). In this direction, the single vectors, the single magnetic forces add up, like people pulling on the same end of a rope.

What we end up with in effect is a magnetic vector in the direction of the external magnetic field (the orange arrow on the z-axis in figure 7); and this vector is a **sum vector** made up by adding the magnetic vectors of the protons pointing upwards.

Now – what does this mean? This means that by placing a patient in the magnet of the MR unit (or in any other strong magnetic field), the patient himself becomes a magnet, i.e. has his own magnetic field. Why? Because the vectors of the protons that do not cancel each other out, add up (figure 8).

As this magnetization is longitudinal to the external magnetic field, it is called **longitudinal magnetization**.

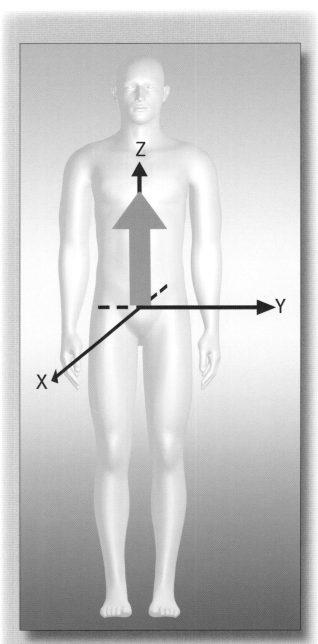

Fig. 8: In a strong external magnetic field, a new magnetic vector is induced in the patient, who becomes a magnet himself. This new magnetic vector is aligned with the external magnetic field.

As we have seen, the resulting new magnetic vector of the patient points in the direction of the external field, along its field lines. This is described as longitudinal direction. And it is actually this new magnetic vector that may be used to get a signal. It would be nice if we could measure this magnetization of the patient, but there is a problem: we cannot measure this magnetic force, as it is in the same direction, parallel to the external magnetic field (figures 7 and 8).

To illustrate this: Imagine that you are sitting on a boat, floating down a river. You have a water hose in your hand and squirt water into the river. For somebody who is watching you from the shore, it is impossible to tell how much water you pour out (i.e. how much new magnetization is added in the old direction).

However, when you point the water hose at the shore, change the direction of the new magnetic field, then the water may perhaps be directly picked up and measured by an impartial observer on the shore (figure 9). What we should learn from this is: magnetization longitudinal to the external magnetic field cannot be measured directly. For this, we need a magnetization which is not longitudinal, but transversal to the external magnetic field.

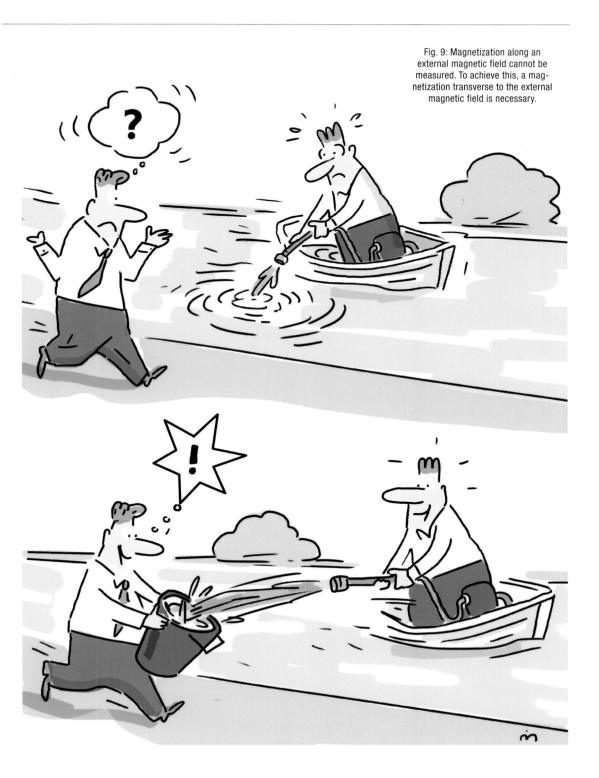

Fig. 9: Magnetization along an external magnetic field cannot be measured. To achieve this, a magnetization transverse to the external magnetic field is necessary.

Time to take a break

Before you walk away, let us just sum up. And when you come back, start out with this summary again.

● Protons have a **positive charge** and possess a spin. Due to this, they have a magnetic field and can be seen as little bar magnets.

● When we put them into a strong external magnetic field, they align with it, some parallel – pointing up –, some anti-parallel – pointing down.

● The protons do not just lie there, but precess around the magnetic field lines. And the stronger the magnetic field, the higher the precession frequency, a relationship that is mathematically described in the Larmor equation.

● Parallel and anti-parallel protons can cancel each others forces out. But as there are more parallel protons on the lower energy level ("pointing up"), we are left with some protons, the magnetic forces of which are not cancelled. All of these protons pointing up, add up their forces in the direction of the external magnetic field. And so when we put the patient in the MR magnet, he has his own magnetic field, which is longitudinal to the external field of the MR machine's magnet (figures 7 and 8). Because it is longitudinal, however, it cannot be measured directly.

What happens after we put the patient into the magnet?

We send in a **radio wave**. The term radio wave is used to describe an electromagnetic wave that is within the frequency range of the waves, which are received by your radio. Well, you can imagine it is not quite like this kind of radio wave. What we actually send into the patient is not a wave of long duration, but a short burst of some **electromagnetic wave**, which is called a **radio frequency- or RF pulse**. The purpose of this RF pulse is to disturb the protons, which are peacefully precessing in alignment with the external magnetic field.

We will hear about the details later. But not every RF pulse disturbs the alignment of the protons: For this, we need a special **RF pulse**, one that can exchange energy with the protons.

This is as if someone were looking at you. You may not notice it, because there is no exchange of energy, so you do not change your position / alignment. However, if someone were to pound you in the stomach, exchange energy with you, your alignment would be disturbed. And this may explain why we need a certain RF pulse that can exchange energy with the protons to change their alignment.

But when can an RF pulse exchange energy with the protons?

For this, it must have the same frequency; the same "speed" as the protons, so to speak. Just imagine that you are driving down a race track on your bike, and someone in the lane next to you wants to hand you a hamburger, i.e. exchange energy with you – as you

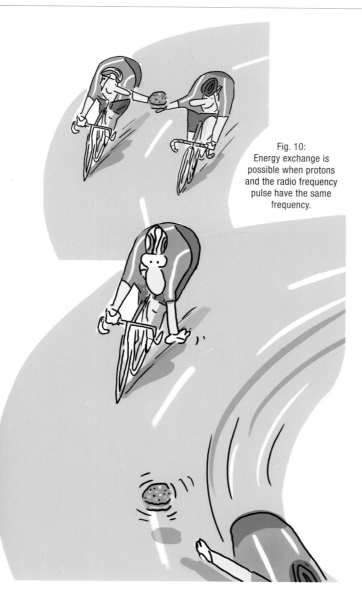

Fig. 10:
Energy exchange is possible when protons and the radio frequency pulse have the same frequency.

are hungry, the hamburger would give you new energy.

This energy transfer is possible when both bikers have the same speed, move around the race track with the same frequency:

With differences in speed/frequency ...

... little or no energy transfer is possible.

The "speed" of protons and resonance

What speed, or better, what frequency did the protons have?

They had their **precession frequency** which can be calculated by the Larmor equation (see page 10). So the **Larmor equation** gives us the necessary frequency of the RF pulse to send in. Only when the RF pulse and the protons have the same frequency, can protons pick up some energy from the radio wave, a phenomenon called **resonance** – this is where the "resonance" in magnetic resonance comes from.

The term resonance can be illustrated by the use of tuning forks. Imagine that you are in a room with different kinds of tuning forks, tuned e.g. to a, e, and d. Somebody enters the room with a tuning fork with "a"-frequency that was struck to emit sound. Of all the tuning forks in the room, all of a sudden the other "a"-forks, and only those, pick up energy, start to vibrate and to emit sound, they show a phenomenon called resonance.

What happens to the protons when exposed to the RF pulse?

Some of them pick up energy, and go from a lower to a higher energy level. Remember, some, which were walking on their feet, start walking on their hands. And this has some effect on the patient's magnetization, as you can see in figure 11. Let us assume that from the net sum of 6 protons pointing up, after the RF pulse is sent in, 2 point down.

The result is that these 2 protons cancel out the magnetic forces of the same number of protons, that point up.

So in effect then, the magnetization in the longitudinal direction – being 6 before the RF pulse – decreases to 2.

What else happens to the protons when exposed to the RF pulse?

As we have just learned, some of the protons pick up energy, and go from a lower to a higher energy level, thus decreasing magnetization in longitudinal direction.

But something else happens. Do you remember what drawings of radio waves look like? Just look at figure 12; they resemble a whip.

And what does a whip make the bears do? It makes them walk in line, in step, in synch – they are in phase.

Believe it or not, the RF pulse also has a whip-like action – not on bears but on protons: When the protons randomly point left/right, back/forth and so on, they also cancel their magnetic forces in these directions (as we read

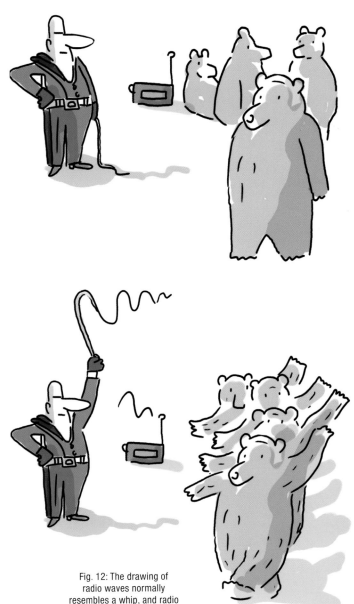

Fig. 12: The drawing of radio waves normally resembles a whip, and radio waves in MRI also have a whip-like action.

Fig. 11: The radio frequency pulse exchanges energy with the protons (A), and some of them are lifted to a higher level of energy, pointing downward in the illustration (B). In effect, the magnetization along the z-axis decreases, as the protons which point down, "neutralize" the same number of protons pointing up.

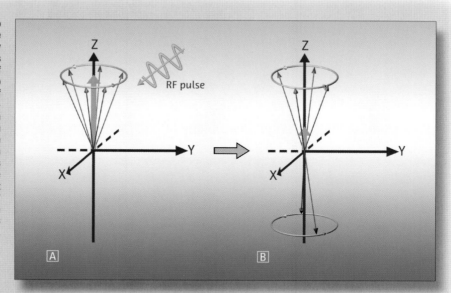

Fig. 13: The radio wave has two effects on the protons: it lifts some protons to a higher level of energy (they point down), and it also causes the protons to precess in step, in phase. The former results in decreasing the magnetization along the z-axis, the so-called longitudinal magnetization. The latter establishes a new magnetization in the x-y-plane (➜), a new transversal magnetization, which moves around with the precessing protons.

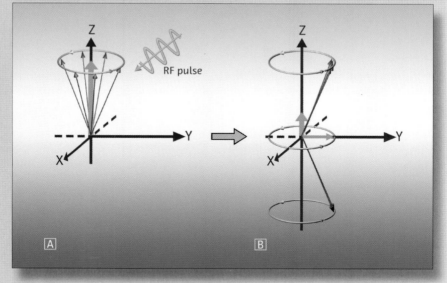

on page 13). Due to the RF pulse, the protons do not point in random directions any more, but move in step, in synch – they are **"in phase"**. They now point in the same direction at the same time, and thus their magnetic vectors add up in this direction. This results in a magnetic vector pointing to the side to which the precessing protons point, and this is in a transverse direction (figure 13). This is why it is called **transversal magnetization**.

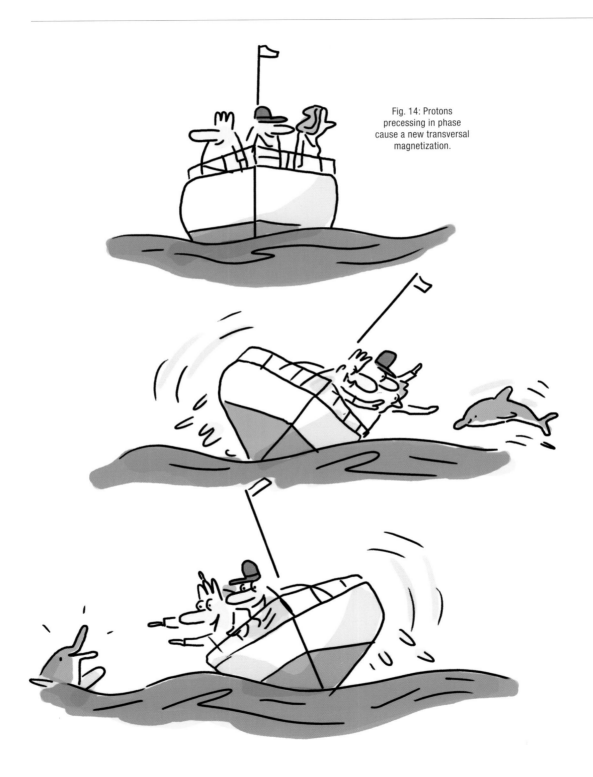

Fig. 14: Protons precessing in phase cause a new transversal magnetization.

So – what were the new things that we have learned?

Repeat them using figure 15.

● When we put the patient in the MR machine, a magnetic field in the patient, longitudinal to the external field, results.

● Sending in an RF pulse that has the same frequency as the precessing frequency of the protons causes two effects:

– Some protons pick up energy, start to walk on their hands, and thus decrease the amount of longitudinal magnetization.

– AND: The protons get in synch, start to precess in phase. Their vectors now also add up in a direction transverse to the external magnetic field, and thus a transversal magnetization is established.

In summary: The RF pulse causes **longitudinal magnetization** to decrease, and establishes a new **transversal magnetization** (figures 13 and 15).

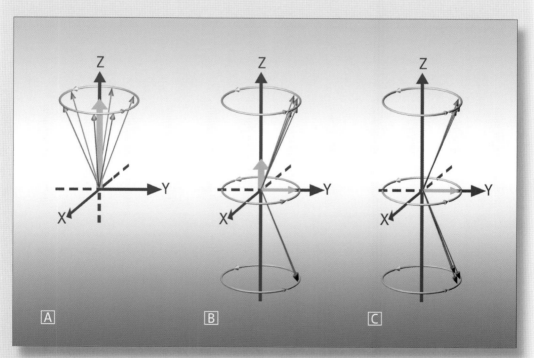

Fig. 15: In a strong external magnetic field, a new magnetic vector along the external field is established in the patient (A). Sending in an RF pulse causes a new transversal magnetization while longitudinal magnetization decreases (B). Depending on the RF pulse, longitudinal magnetization may even totally disappear (C).

The transversal vector – a closer look

Let us have a look at the newly established transversal magnetization vector.

This moves in phase with the precessing protons (figure 16). The new magnetic vector comes towards you, goes away from you, comes again towards you, and so on.

And this is important: the **magnetic vector**, by constantly moving, constantly changing, induces an electric current. We have talked about the opposite already: the moving electrical charge of the proton, the electric current, induces the proton's magnetic field. This also is true the other way around: a moving magnetic field causes an electrical current, e.g. in an antenna. And this electrical current induced by the moving magnetic field is the MRI signal. As the transversal magnetic vector moves around with the precessing protons, it moves with the precession frequency. The resulting MR signal therefore also has the **precession frequency** (figure 16): But ... how can we make a picture out of this electrical current, which is actually our MR signal?

For this we have to know, where in the body the signal came from. How can we know that? The trick is really quite simple: we do not put the patient into a **magnetic field** which has the same strength all over the section of the patient, which we want to examine.

Instead we take a magnetic field, which has a different strength at each

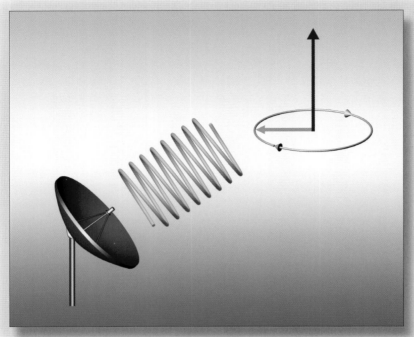

Fig. 16: The new transversal magnetization moves around with the precessing protons (see figure 13). Thus for an external observer, transversal magnetization constantly changes its direction, and can induce a signal in an antenna.

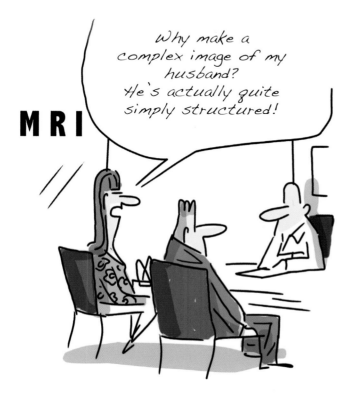

signal from different locations also has a different frequency. And by the frequency we can assign a signal to a certain location.

It is like with your TV: when you are in the kitchen (where you probably do not have a TV) and hear a sound from your favorite TV show, you know where the sound is coming from. It comes from the spot in your apartment where the TV stands. What you subconsciously do, is to connect a certain sound to a certain location in space.

That is enough about spatial information for now, we will go into more detail about this on page 87.

Further details about the MR signal

If our protons rotated around **in synch**, in phase, and nothing changes, then we would get a signal as illustrated in figure 16.

This, however, is not what happens. As soon as the RF pulse is switched off, the whole system, which was disturbed by the RF pulse, goes back to its original quiet, peaceful state, it relaxes.

The newly established transverse magnetization starts to disappear – a process called **transversal relaxation**, and the longitudinal magnetization grows back to its original size – a process called **longitudinal relaxation**.

Why is that?

The reason why the longitudinal magnetization grows back to its normal size is easier to explain, so let us start with that (see figure 17).

No proton walks on its hands longer than it has to – a sort of human trait. The protons that were lifted onto a higher energy level by the RF pulse go back to their lower energy level, and start to walk on their feet again.

point of the patient's cross-section. What does this do?

We have heard that the precession frequency of a proton depends on the strength of the magnetic field – as the frequency of a violin string depends on the strength with which you pull it.

If this strength differs from point to point in the patient, then protons in different places precess with different frequencies. And as they precess with different frequencies, the resulting MR

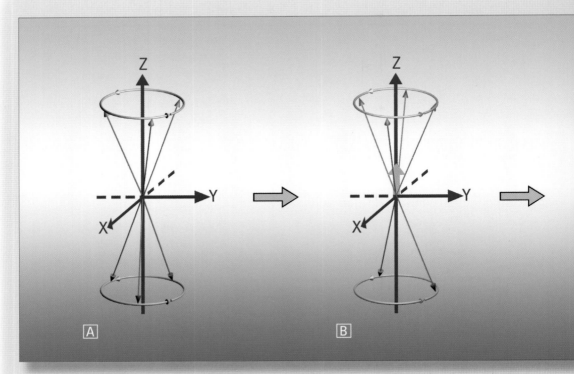

Fig. 17: After the RF pulse is switched off, protons go back from their higher to the lower state of energy, i.e. point up again. This is illustrated "one-by-one". The effect is that longitudinal magnetization increases and grows back to its original value. Note that for simplicity the protons were not depicted as being in phase: this subject is covered in more detail in figures 20 and 26.

After the RF pulse is switched off, protons go back to the lower state of energy, i.e. point up again, but not all protons do this at exactly the same time. Instead it is a continuous process, as if one proton after the other goes back to its original state. This is illustrated in figure 17 for a group of protons. The effect is that **longitudinal magnetization** increases and grows back to its original value.

What happens to the energy which they had picked up from the RF pulse?

This energy is just handed over to their surroundings, the so-called **lattice**.

And this is why this process is not only called longitudinal relaxation, but also **spin-lattice relaxation**.

By going back on their feet, pointing upwards again, these protons no longer cancel out the magnetic vectors of the same number of protons pointing up, as they did before. So, the magnetization in this direction, the **longitudinal magnetization** increases, and finally goes back to its original value (figure 17).

If you plot the longitudinal magnetization vs. time after the RF pulse is switched off, you get a curve like figure 18. It increases with time. This curve is also called a T_1-**curve**.

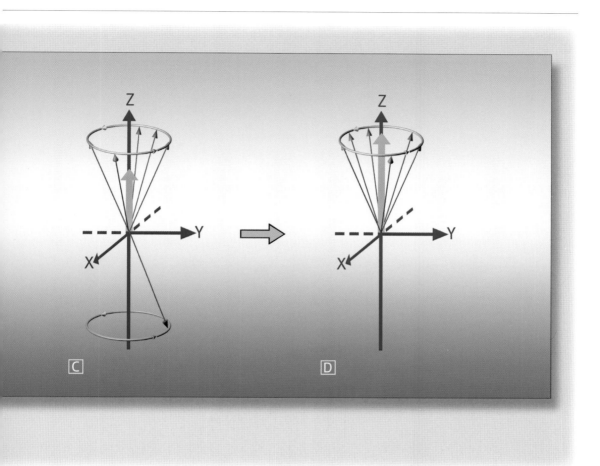

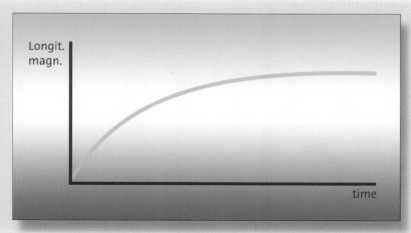

Fig. 18: If one plots the longitudinal magnetization vs. time after the RF pulse was switched off, one gets a so-called T_1-curve.

The time that it takes for the longitudinal magnetization to recover, to go back to its original value, is described by the **longitudinal relaxation time**, also called T_1. This actually is not the exact time it takes, but a time constant, describing how fast this process goes.

This is like taking time for one circuit round at a car race.

The time gives you an idea of how long the race may take, but not the exact time. Or more scientifically, T_1 is a time constant comparable to the time constants that for example describe radioactive decay.

That T_1 is the **longitudinal relaxation time**, can easily be remembered:

If you turn the "1" upside down, it looks very much like an "l" as in longitudinal.

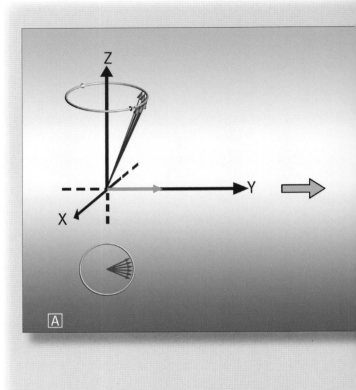

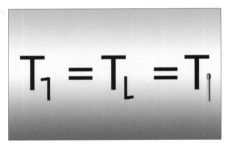

Fig. 19: T_1 is the longitudinal relaxation time that has something to do with the exchange of thermal energy.

Reminding you also that it describes the spin-"1"attice relaxation.

But there are more hidden hints to this: the "1" also looks like a match. And this match should remind you of something, which we also have mentioned already: longitudinal relaxation has something to do with exchange of energy, thermal energy, which the protons emit to the surrounding lattice while returning to their lower state of energy.

About T_2

Enough about the longitudinal magnetization – what happens with the transversal magnetization?

Let us assume that this is the situation just before the RF pulse is switched off.

When the RF pulse is switched off, the protons get out of step, out of phase again, as nobody is telling them to stay in step. For the sake of simplicity, this has been illustrated for a group of protons which all "point up" in figure 20. We heard earlier that protons precess with a frequency

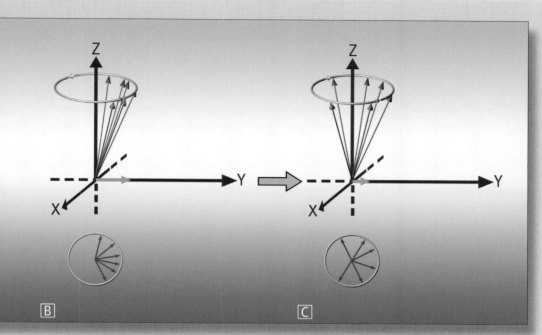

Fig. 20: After the RF pulse is switched off, protons lose phase coherence, they get out of step. When you look at these dephasing proton ensembles from the top (which is illustrated in the lower part of the figure), it becomes obvious, how they fan out. Fanning out, they point less and less in the same direction, and thus transversal magnetization decreases.

which is determined by the magnetic field strength that they are in. And all the protons should experience the same magnetic field. This, however, is not the case:

Firstly, the field of the MR magnet, in which the patient is placed, is not totally uniform, not totally homogeneous, but varies a little, thus causing different precession frequencies.

Secondly, each proton is influenced by the small magnetic fields from neighboring nuclei that are also not distributed evenly, thus causing different precession frequencies, too. These internal magnetic field variations are somehow characteristic of a tissue. So, after the RF pulse is switched off, the protons are no longer forced to stay in step; and as they have different precession frequencies – as we have just learned – they will be soon out of phase.

It is interesting to see how fast the protons get out of phase: just suppose that one proton – p1 – is rotating at 10 million revolutions per second, i.e. with a precessing frequency of 10 megahertz.

Due to inhomogeneities, a neighboring proton – p2 – is in a magnetic field, which is 1% stronger; this proton has a precession frequency of 10.1 megahertz, 1% more. In 5 microseconds (0.000005 sec or 5×10^{-6}), p2 will have made 50.5 turns or revolutions, while proton p1 will have made only 50. So in this short time span, the protons will be 180° out of phase, cancelling their magnetic moments in the respective plane.

Similar to what we did for the longitudinal magnetization, we can plot transversal magnetization versus time. What we get is a curve like in figure 21. This curve is going downhill, as **transversal magnetization** disappears with time. And as you probably expect: there is also a time constant, describing how fast transversal magnetization vanishes, goes downhill. This time constant is the **transversal relaxation time** T_2.

How to remember, what "T_2" is? Easy:

T_2 is T x 2 is TT is Tt

and this means, it describes the "T transversal", thus the relaxation of the transversal magnetization. The resulting curve in figure 21 thus is called a T_2**-curve**. Another term for transversal relaxation is **spin-spin-relaxation**, reminding us of the underlying mechanism, a spin-spin interaction. How to remember which one is the T_1- and which the T_2-curve? Just put both curves together. You can see something like a mountain with a ski slope. You first have to climb to the top – T_1-curve – before you ski down – T_2-curve (figure 22).

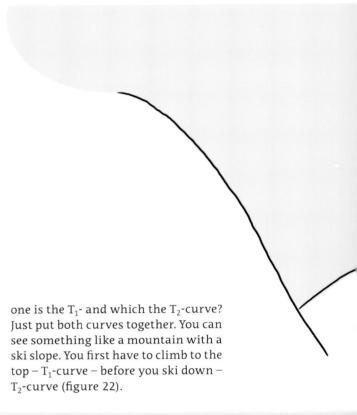

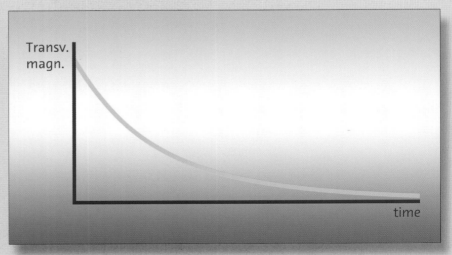

Fig. 21: If one plots transversal magnetization vs. time after the RF pulse is switched off, one gets a curve as illustrated, which is called a T_2-curve.

Transv. magn.

time

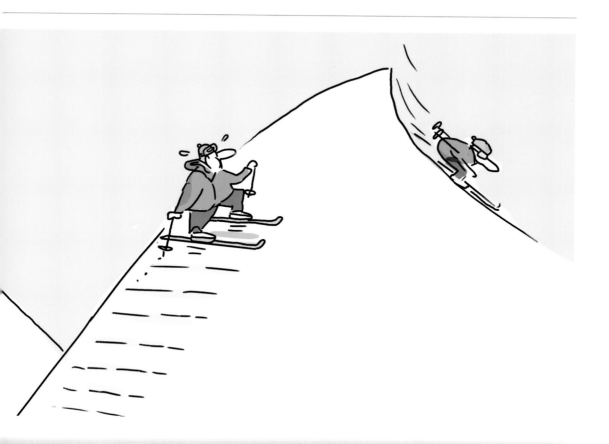

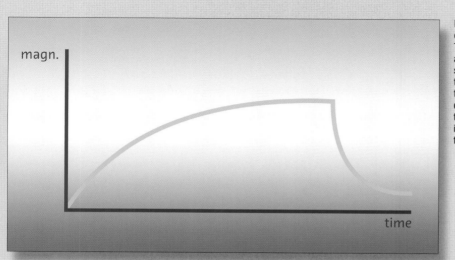

Fig. 22: Coupling of a T_1- and a T_2-curve resembles a mountain with a slope. It takes longer to climb a mountain than to slide or jump down, which helps to remember that T_1 is normally longer than T_2.

So, time for a review

We have learned:
- Protons are like little magnets.
- In an external magnetic field, they align parallel or anti-parallel.
- The lower energy state – parallel – is preferred, so a few more protons align this way.
- The protons perform a motion that resembles the wobbling of a spinning top.
- This motion is called precession.
- The precession frequency is dependent on the strength of the external magnetic field – a relationship which is described by the Larmor equation. The stronger the magnetic field, the higher the precession frequency.
- Protons "pointing" in opposite directions cancel each other's magnetic effects in the respective directions.
- As there are more protons aligned parallel to the external field, there is a net magnetic moment aligned with or longitudinal to the external magnetic field.
- A radio frequency pulse that has the same frequency as the precessing protons, can cause resonance, transfer energy to the protons. This results in more protons being anti-parallel and thus neutralizing or cancelling more protons in the opposite direction. Consequence: the longitudinal magnetization decreases.
- The RF pulse also causes the protons to precess in synch, in phase. This results in a new magnetic vector, the transversal magnetization, which moves around with the precessing protons.
- When the RF pulse is switched off,
  – transversal magnetization decreases and disappears,
  – while longitudinal magnetization increases again.

This longitudinal relaxation is described by a time constant T_1, the **longitudinal relaxation time**.
The transversal relaxation is described by a time constant T_2, the **transversal relaxation time**.
Longitudinal and transversal relaxation are different, independent processes, and that is why we discussed them individually (see figures 17 and 20).
This is what you should know by now.

How long is a relaxation time?

At the end of our last section we already learned that it takes longer to climb a mountain than to ski down, which means that T_1 is normally longer than T_2.

Just to give you an idea: T_1 is about 2–10 times as long as T_2. Or in absolute terms in biological tissues: T_1 is about 300 to 2,000 msec, and T_2 is about 30 to 150 msec.

It is difficult to pinpoint the end of the longitudinal and transversal relaxation exactly. Thus, T_1 and T_2 were not defined as the time when relaxation has completed. Instead T_1 was defined as the time when about 63% of the original longitudinal magnetization was reached.

T_2 is the time, when transversal magnetization decreased to 37% of the original value. These percentages are derived from mathematical equations ($63\% = 1 - 1/e$; $37\% = 1/e$) describing signal intensity, but we do not want to go into more detail here. (However, we should mention that $1/T_1$ is also called **longitudinal relaxation rate**, and $1/T_2$ **transversal relaxation rate**.)

Previously, it was believed that measuring the relaxation times would give tissue characteristic results, and thus enable exact tissue typing. This, however, proved to be wrong, as there is quite an overlap of time ranges. What is a long, what is a short relaxation time, and which tissues have long or short relaxation times?

Look at figure 23 – what do you see? You see somebody having a long drink, something liquid (representing water). When you go to your favorite bar, which is naturally crowded, as it is a popular place, and order a long drink, you have to wait quite a while to get your drink – T_1 is long. When you finally have your long drink, it also takes you a long time to drink it, so T_2 is also long. And we want to remember: water/liquids have a long T_1 and a long T_2.

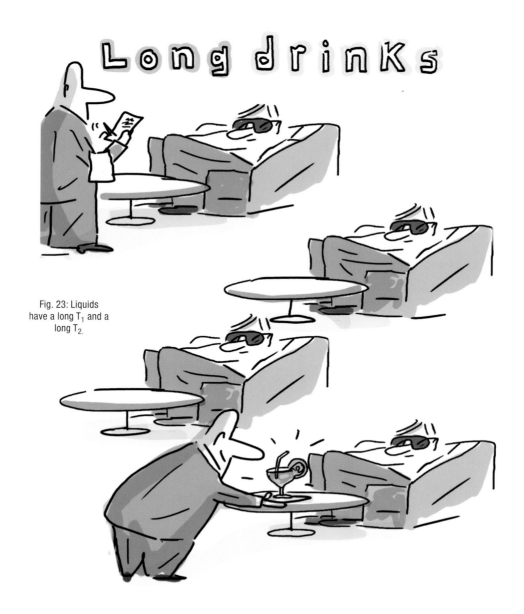

Fig. 23: Liquids have a long T_1 and a long T_2.

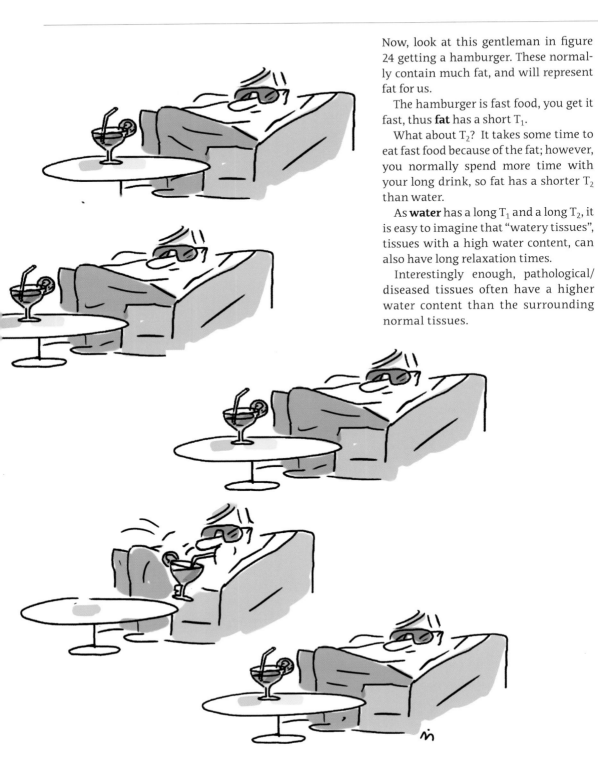

Now, look at this gentleman in figure 24 getting a hamburger. These normally contain much fat, and will represent fat for us.

The hamburger is fast food, you get it fast, thus **fat** has a short T_1.

What about T_2? It takes some time to eat fast food because of the fat; however, you normally spend more time with your long drink, so fat has a shorter T_2 than water.

As **water** has a long T_1 and a long T_2, it is easy to imagine that "watery tissues", tissues with a high water content, can also have long relaxation times.

Interestingly enough, pathological/diseased tissues often have a higher water content than the surrounding normal tissues.

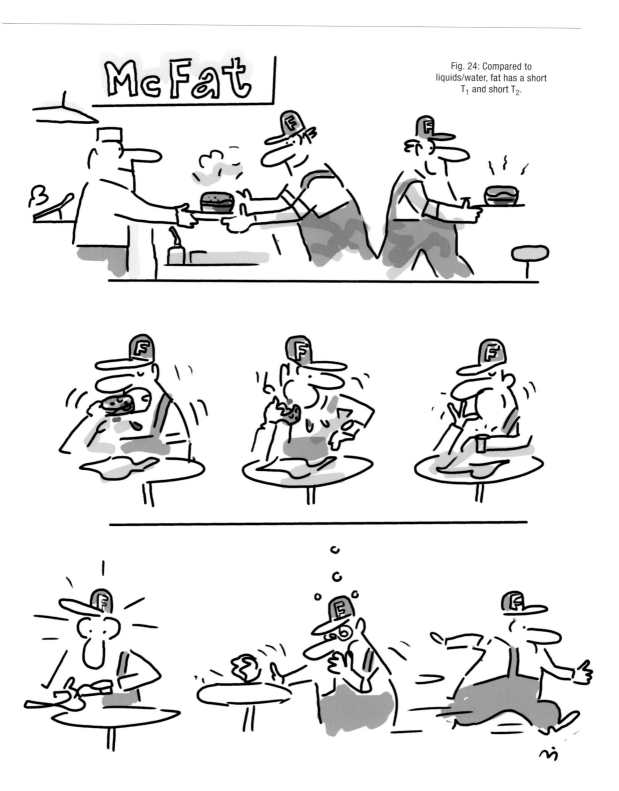

Fig. 24: Compared to liquids/water, fat has a short T_1 and short T_2.

What is T_1 influenced by?

Actually, T_1 depends on tissue composition, structure and surroundings.

As we have learned, **T_1-relaxation** has something to do with the exchange of thermal energy, which is handed over from the protons to the surroundings, the lattice. The precessing protons have a magnetic field that constantly changes directions, and which constantly fluctuates according to the Larmor frequency. The lattice also has its own magnetic fields.

The protons now want to hand energy over to the lattice to relax.

This can be done very effectively, when the fluctuations of the magnetic fields in the lattice occur with a frequency that is near the to Larmor frequency.

When the lattice consists of pure liquid/water, it is difficult for the protons to get rid of their energy, as the small water molecules move too rapidly.

And as the protons, which are on the higher energy level, cannot hand their energy over to the lattice quickly, they will only slowly go back to their lower energy level, their longitudinal alignment.

Thus it takes a long time for the longitudinal magnetization to show up again, and this means that liquids/water have long T_1s.

When the lattice consists of medium-size molecules – most body tissues can be looked at as liquids containing various-sized molecules, kind of like a soup – that move and have fluctuating magnetic fields near the Larmor frequency of the precessing protons, energy can be transferred much faster, thus T_1 is short.

This can again be illustrated by our hamburger and bicycle example: (see page 17) handing over hamburgers – i.e.

energy – from one bicycle – proton – to the other – lattice – is easy and efficient, when both move with the same speed. With a difference in speed, the energy transfer will be less efficient.

Why does fat have a short T_1?

The carbon bonds at the ends of the fatty acids have frequencies near the Larmor frequency, thus resulting in effective energy transfer.

And why is T_1 longer in stronger magnetic fields?

As we heard in the beginning, the precession frequency depends on magnetic field strength, a relationship described by the Larmor equation.

If we have a stronger magnetic field, then the protons precess faster.

And when they precess faster, they have more problems handing down their energy to a lattice with more slowly fluctuating magnetic fields.

What influences T_2?

T_2-relaxation comes about when protons get out of phase, which – as we already know – has two causes: inhomogeneities of the external magnetic field, and inhomogeneities of the local magnetic fields within the tissues (see page 27). As water molecules move around very fast, their local magnetic fields fluctuate fast, and therefore kind of average each other out, so there are no big net differences in internal magnetic fields from place to place. And if there are no big differences in magnetic field strength within a tissue, the protons stay in step for a long time, before they dephase, and so T_2 is longer. With impure liquids, e.g. those containing some larger molecules, there are bigger variations in the local magnetic fields. The larger molecules do not move around as fast, so their local magnetic fields do not cancel each other out as much. These larger differences in local magnetic fields consequently cause larger differences in precessing frequencies, thus protons get out of phase faster, T_2 is shorter.

This can be illustrated by the following example: imagine that you drive down a street with many pot holes. When you drive slowly (which is equal to the surroundings moving slowly and you are standing still), you will be bumping up and down in your car as it drives over each pot hole. The differ-

ences in the surroundings (the magnetic field variations) influence you considerably. When you drive very fast (which is the same as if the surroundings move very fast), you do not feel each single pot hole anymore. Before they have a major effect on you, you are already back at normal street level; thus their effect is averaged out, you are much less influenced by differences in the surroundings (the variations in magnetic field strength).

What does all this have to do with what we want to know? All these processes influence how your MR picture will finally look!

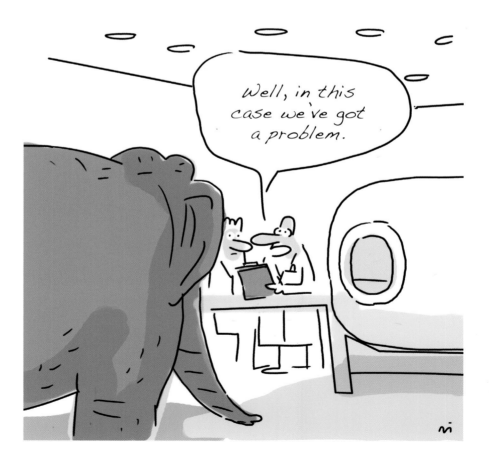

A brief review might be advisable:

- T_1 is longer than T_2.
- T_1 varies with the magnetic field strength; in stronger magnetic fields it is longer.
- Water has a long T_1, fat has a short T_1.
- T_2 of water is longer than the T_2 of impure liquids containing larger molecules.

An experiment ...

Now let us perform an experiment

Look at figure 25, where you can see two protons, precessing around the z-axis. I hope you recall that the z-axis indicates the direction of a magnetic field line (see page 9). Instead of only these two protons, in reality there may be 8 pointing up and 6 pointing down, or 82 up and 80 down – there

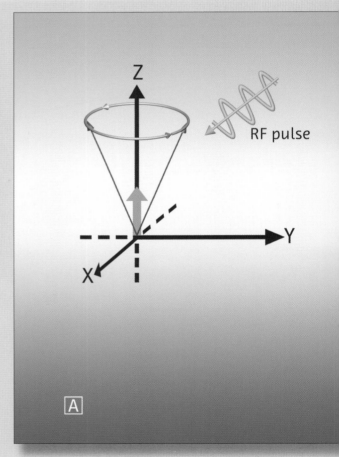

Fig. 25: If after the RF pulse the number of protons on the higher energy level equals the number of protons on the lower energy, longitudinal magnetization has disappeared, and there is only transversal magnetization due to phase coherence. The magnetic vector seems to have been "tilted" 90° to the side. The corresponding RF pulse is thus also called a 90° pulse.

shall only be two more protons pointing up.

As we know, these are the ones that have a net magnetic effect because their effects are not cancelled out.

Now let us send in an RF pulse, which has just the correct strength and duration, so that one of the two protons picks up energy to go into a higher state of energy, i.e. points down/walks on its hands.

What will happen? The **longitudinal magnetization** (up to now resulting from two protons pointing up)

will decrease, in our example to zero (one pointing up is neutralized by one pointing down). But: as both protons are in phase, there is now a transversal magnetization which had not been there before.

The RF pulse seemingly "tilts" the longitudinal **magnetic vector** 90° to the side.

Such an RF pulse is called a **90° pulse**. Naturally, other RF pulses are also possible, and are named accordingly, e.g. **180° pulse**.

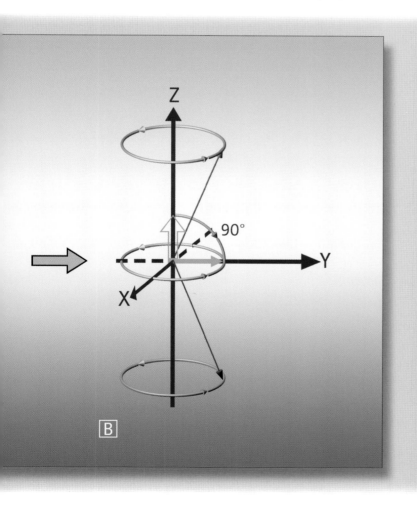

To really understand this, let us look at another example. In figure 26A, we have 6 protons pointing up; we send in an RF pulse, which lifts 3 of them onto a higher energy level (B).

The result: we no longer have a longitudinal, but a transversal magnetization (again having used a 90° pulse).

What happens, when the RF pulse is switched off?

Two things happen: protons go back to their lower state of energy, and they lose **phase coherence**.

It is important to note that both processes occur simultaneously and independently. For the sake of simplicity, let us look at what happens step by step, and first focus on the **longitudinal magnetization**:

● After the RF pulse is switched off (figure 26C), one proton goes back to the lower energy state, result-

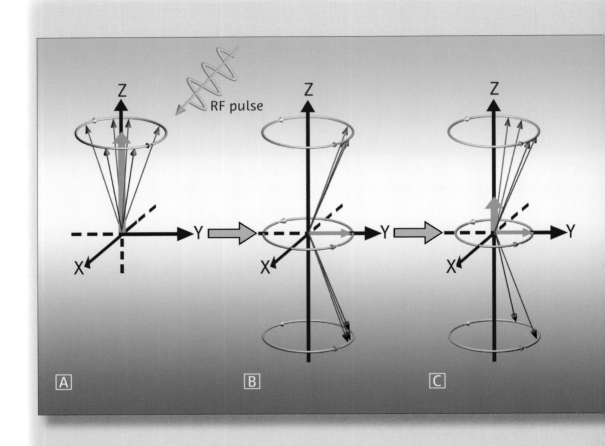

ing in 4 protons pointing up, and two pointing down. The net effect: we now have a longitudinal magnetization of "2".

● Then the next proton goes back up; now 5 protons are pointing up, and one down, resulting in a net longitudinal magnetization of "4" (figure 26D).

● After the next proton goes up, longitudinal magnetization equals "6" (figure 26E).

You surely have already noticed that the transversal magnetization decreases at the same time (figure 26C-E). Why? You should be able to answer this: After the RF pulse is switched off, the precessing protons lose phase coherence.

In figure 26B, all protons point in the same direction, but then increasingly get out of phase, and thus kind of fan out (figure 26C-E).

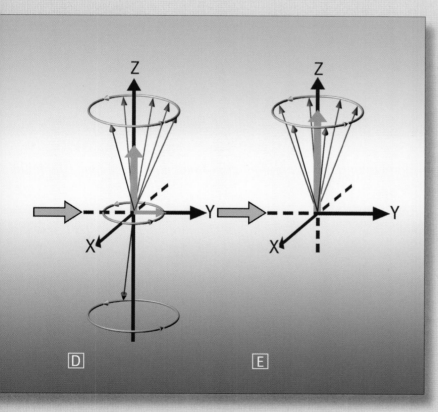

Fig. 26: (A) shows the situation before and (B) immediately after an RF pulse is sent in. The RF pulse causes the longitudinal magnetization (↑) to decrease, and with a 90° pulse as illustrated, it becomes zero (B). Protons also start to precess in phase (B), which causes the new transversal magnetization (→). After the RF pulse is switched off (C-E), longitudinal magnetization increases, recovers, and transversal magnetization disappears, decays. Both processes are due to entirely different mechanisms and occur independently, even though at the same time.

In figure 27, only the longitudinal and transversal **magnetic vectors** are depicted at corresponding times as in figure 26. These magnetic vectors add up to a sum vector (→).

As you remember, vectors represent forces of a certain size and a certain direction. If you add up vectors pointing to different directions, you will come up with a direction that is somewhere in between, depending on the amount of force in the original directions. If we do the same with the longitudinal and the transversal vector, we get the **sum vector**.

This sum vector is very important, as it represents the total magnetic moment of a tissue in general, and thus can be used instead of the two single vectors, representing longitudinal and transversal magnetization separately. Our magnetic sum vector during relax-

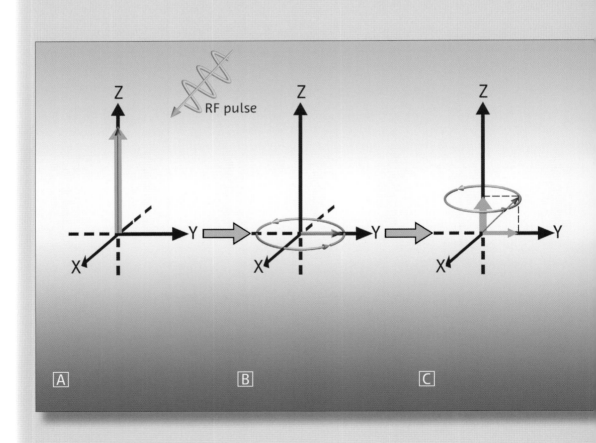

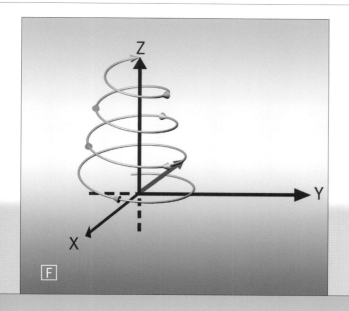

ation goes back to a longitudinal direction, in the end equaling the **longitudinal magnetization**.

What we have to remember is that this whole system is actually precessing, including the sum magnetic vector. And thus – after the RF pulse is switched off – the sum vector will actually perform a spiraling motion (figure 27F).

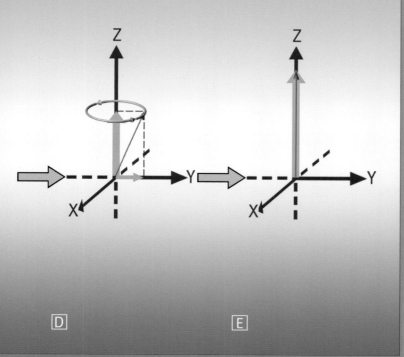

Fig. 27: In this illustration only the longitudinal and transversal magnetization vectors from our experiment in figure 26 are depicted. In (A) – before the RF pulse – there is only longitudinal magnetization. Immediately after the 90° RF pulse there is no longitudinal but new transversal magnetization (B), and this transversal magnetization vector is spinning around. With time this transversal magnetization decreases, while longitudinal magnetization increases (C-D), until the starting point with no transversal but full longitudinal magnetization is reached again (E). Transversal and longitudinal magnetization vectors add up to a sum vector (→). This sum vector performs a spiraling motion (F) when it changes its direction from being in the transversal (x-y) plane (no longitudinal magnetization) to its final position along the z-axis (no transversal magnetization).

I hope that you recall that a changing magnetic force/moment can induce an electric current, which is the signal that we receive and use in MR.

So if we put up an antenna somewhere (figure 28), we will get a signal as illustrated. This is easy to imagine, if you think of the antenna as a micro-phone, and the sum magnetic vector as having some kind of a sound-emitting device like a steam pipe at its tip. The further the vector goes away from the microphone, the less loud the sound. The frequency of the sound, however, remains the same because the **sum vector** spins with the precessing frequency

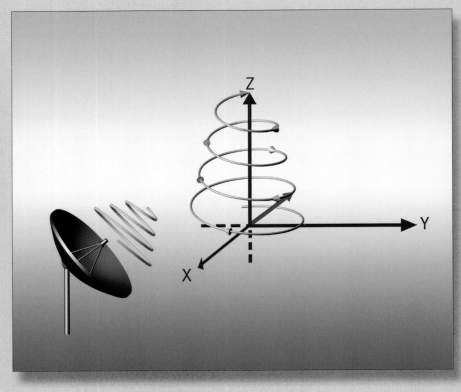

Fig. 28: For an external observer, the sum vector of figure 27F constantly changes its direction and magnitude, while it performs its spiraling motion. The sum vector induces an electrical current in an antenna, the MR signal. This is of greatest magnitude, immediately after the RF pulse is switched off, and then decreases.

(figure 29). So the signal from our experiment disappears with time, however, it has a constant frequency.

This type of signal is called a **free induction decay** signal, or **FID signal**.

By now it should be obvious that the magnetic vector directly determines the MRI signal and signal intensity by inducing electrical currents in the antenna. Instead of the terms "longitudinal" or "transversal magnetization", we can also use the term "signal or signal intensity" at the axis of our T_1- and T_2-curves.

This will hopefully become clearer, as you continue reading.

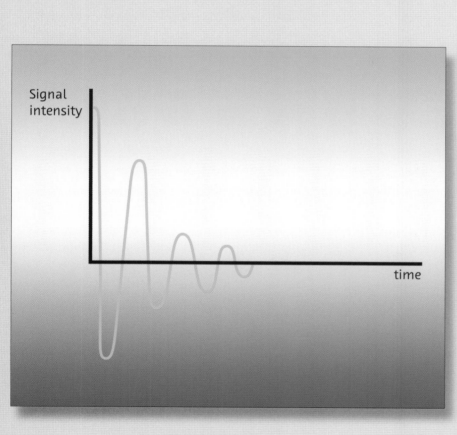

Signal intensity

time

Fig. 29: The signal from our experiment in figures 26 to 28 disappears with time, however, it has a constant frequency. This type of signal is called a FID (free induction decay) signal.

Another experiment

Let us perform another experiment similar to the one illustrated in figure 30. As we want to concentrate purely on the magnetization, we can leave out the coordinate system. In figure 30A, we have two tissues, A and B, which have different relaxation times as we will see later. We send in a 90° RF pulse, switch it off and wait a certain time TR_{long} (we will explain later, why we use the term **TR**). Then we send in a second 90° pulse. What will happen?

As after the time TR_{long} tissue A and tissue B have regained all of their **longitudinal magnetization** (frame 5), the **transversal magnetization** after the second pulse will be the same for both tissues, as it was after the first RF pulse (frame 1). Tissue A cannot be differentiated from tissue B.

What if we do not wait so long from pulse to pulse? Let us look at figure 30B:

After the first pulse, an equally sized transversal magnetization is established in both tissues, which decreases after the pulse is switched off. At TR_{short} however, tissue A has regained more of its longitudinal magnetization than tissue B. When the second 90° pulse now "tilts" the longitudinal magnetization 90 degrees, the transversal magnetic vector of tissue A is larger than that of tissue B.

And when this vector of A is larger, it will reach closer to our antenna; thus the imaginary steam pipe at the tip of vector A will cause a louder, stronger signal in our "microphone", the antenna, than the vector of B.

The difference in signal intensity in this experiment depends on the difference in longitudinal magnetization, and this means on the difference in T_1 between the tissues. Using these two pulses, we can now differentiate tissue A from tissue B, which in our experiment was impossible, choosing only one 90° pulse or two 90° pulses that are a long time apart (after a long time, the differences in T_1 between tissue A and B no longer play a role in our experiment, because after that time the tissue B with the longer T_1 is back to its original state, too).

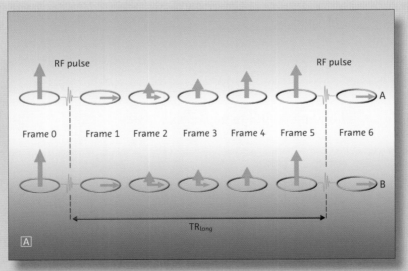

Fig. 30A

When we do not wait as long as in figure 30A, but send in the RF pulse after a shorter time (TR_{short}), like in figure 30B, longitudinal magnetization of tissue B, which has the longer T_1, has not recovered as much as that of tissue A with the shorter T_1. The transversal magnetization

When you use more than one RF pulse – a succession of RF pulses – you use a so-called **pulse sequence**. As you can use different pulses, e.g. 90° or 180° pulses, and the time intervals between successive pulses can be different, there can be many different pulse sequences. As we saw in our experiment, the choice of a pulse sequence will determine, what kind of signal you get out of a tissue. So it is necessary to carefully choose and also describe the pulse sequence for a specific study.

The pulse sequence that we used was made up of one type of pulse only, the 90° pulse. This was repeated after a certain time, which is called **TR = time to repeat**.

How did TR influence the signal in our experiment?

With a long TR we got similar signals from both tissues, both would appear the same on an MR picture, since the transversal magnetization was the same for both tissues. Using a shorter TR, there was a difference in signal intensity between the tissues, determined by their difference in T_1.

The resulting image is called a T_1**-weighted image**. This means that the difference of signal intensity between tissues in that image, the **tissue contrast**, is mainly due to their difference in T_1. However, there is always more than one parameter influencing the tissue contrast; in our example, T_1 is just the most outstanding one.

What is a short, what is a long TR?

A **TR** of less than 500 msec is considered to be short, a TR greater than 1,500 msec to be long. As you may imagine or know already, we cannot only create T_1**-weighted images**, but also T_2**-weighted images**, and so-called **proton density (-weighted) images**.

This **proton density**, which is also called **spin density**, influences tissue contrast and can be explained quite simply: where there are many protons, we will have "lots" of signals. Where there are no protons, there will be no signal. We will read more about this later. The point is that by using certain pulse sequences, we can make certain tissue characteristics to be more or less important in the resulting image.

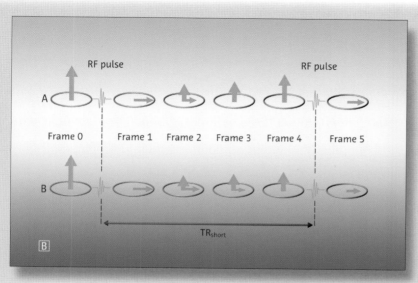

Fig. 30B

of the two tissues after the second RF pulse will then be different (frame 5). Thus, by changing the time between successive RF pulses, we can influence and modify magnetization and the signal intensity of tissues.

By choosing a pulse sequence, the doctor can be compared to a conductor of an orchestra (figure 31): he can influence the overall appearance of the sound (signal) by making certain instruments (parameters) influence the sound more than others. All instruments (parameters), however, always play some role in the final sound (signal).

Let us go back to our experiment once more for a short repetition:

● With a certain type of RF pulse, we can cause the longitudinal magnetization to disappear, while a transversal magnetization appears. The "net magnetization" (the sum vector of longitudinal and transversal magnetization) is "tilted" 90° in this case (when we started, we only had longitudinal magnetization). The corresponding RF pulse is therefore called a 90° pulse.

● The transversal component of the net magnetization can induce a measurable signal in an antenna.

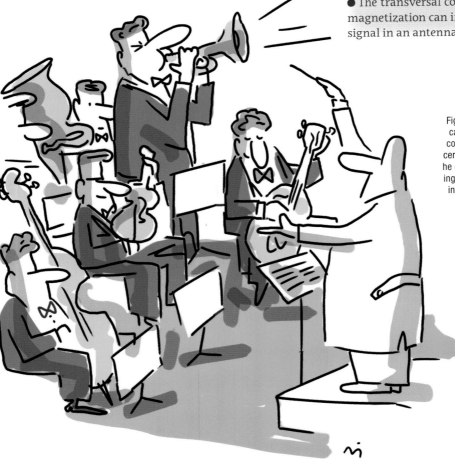

Fig. 31: The MRI doctor can be compared to a conductor: by choosing certain pulse sequences, he can modify the resulting signal, which is itself influenced by different parameters.

● Immediately after the RF pulse relaxation begins: transversal magnetization starts to disappear and longitudinal relaxation begins to reappear. The signal disappears.

● When we send in the second 90° pulse, the net magnetization is again tilted 90°, and we again receive a signal.

● The strength of this signal depends (among other things) on the amount of longitudinal magnetization we start out with. Do you remember the T_1-curve? The T_1-curve described the relationship between time (after an RF pulse) and the amount of longitudinal magnetization (figure 18).

When we wait a long time before sending in our second RF pulse, longitudinal magnetization will have recovered totally.

The signal after the second RF pulse will thus be the same as the one after the first pulse. However, when the second pulse comes in earlier, the signal will be different, since the amount of longitudinal magnetization at that time is less.

The difference in signal intensity

In figure 32, you can see the T_1-curves for brain and for cerebrospinal fluid (CSF). Brain has a shorter longitudinal relaxation time than CSF.

At the time 0, we have no longitudinal magnetization at all, and this can be the time immediately after our first 90° pulse. When we wait a long time before we repeat the 90° pulse (TR_{long}), **longitudinal magnetization** has pretty much recovered. The longitudinal magnetic vectors that will be "tilted" 90°, differ only to a small degree, so there will only be a small difference in signal intensity, i.e. tissue contrast between brain and CSF is small. If we, however, send in the second pulse after a shorter time, TR_{short}, the difference in longitudinal magnetization is rather large, so there will be a better **tissue contrast**.

And as we can see from the distance between the two curves, there is a time span where tissue contrast is most pronounced.

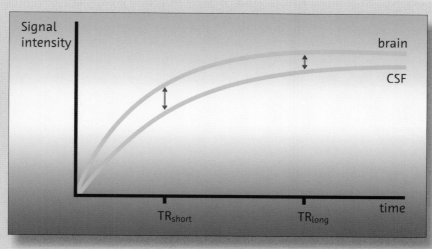

Fig. 32: Brain has a shorter longitudinal relaxation time than CSF. With a short TR, the signal intensities of brain and CSF differ more than after a long TR.

Why are the signals after a very long time TR between pulses not identical?

We have heard the explanation already. The signal intensity depends on many parameters. When we wait a long time, T_1 does not influence the tissue contrast any more, however, there may still be a possible difference in the **proton density** of the tissues in question.

And when we wait a very long time, TR in our experiment from figure 32, the difference in signal is mainly due to different proton densities, we have a so-called **proton density-** (or **spin density-**) **weighted image**.

Now we have heard about T_1- and proton density-weighted images.

T₂-weighted images

How do we obtain a T₂-weighted image?

This is a little more difficult to understand. Let us perform another experiment, which is a little different from the ones before. First, we use a 90° pulse. The longitudinal magnetization is tilted, we get a transversal magnetization. What happens after this pulse, when we wait a short time?

You can surely answer this question without difficulty – if not, go back to page 27 before you continue to read.

After the pulse is switched off, longitudinal magnetization starts to reappear, the transversal magnetization, however, starts to disappear. Why does the transversal magnetization disappear? It is because the pro-

tons . . . lose phase coherence, as we learned earlier.

This is illustrated in figure 33 for three protons, which are almost exactly in phase as seen in (A) but increasingly spread out, as they have different precession frequencies (see B and C). The loss of **phase coherence** results in decreasing transversal magnetization and thus loss of signal. Now we will do something new: af-

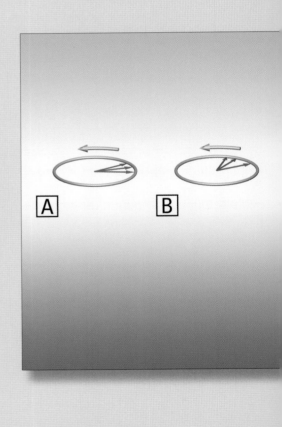

ter a certain time (which we call TE/2, half of **TE**, for reasons you will understand in a few minutes), we will send in a **180° pulse**. What happens?

The 180° pulse acts like a rubber wall; it makes the protons turn around, so that they precess in exactly the opposite direction, which is clockwise.

The result is that the faster precessing protons are now behind the slow-

er ones. If we wait another time TE/2, the faster ones will have caught up with the slower ones (see figure 33F).

At this point in time, the protons are nearly in phase again, which results in a stronger transversal magnetization, and thus in a stronger signal again. A little later, however, the faster precessing protons will be ahead again, with the signal decreasing again.

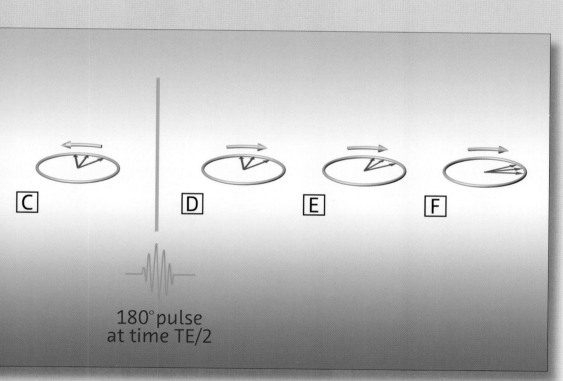

180° pulse
at time TE/2

Fig. 33: After the RF pulse is switched off, the protons dephase (A-C). The 180° pulse causes them to precess in the opposite direction, and so they rephase again (D-F).

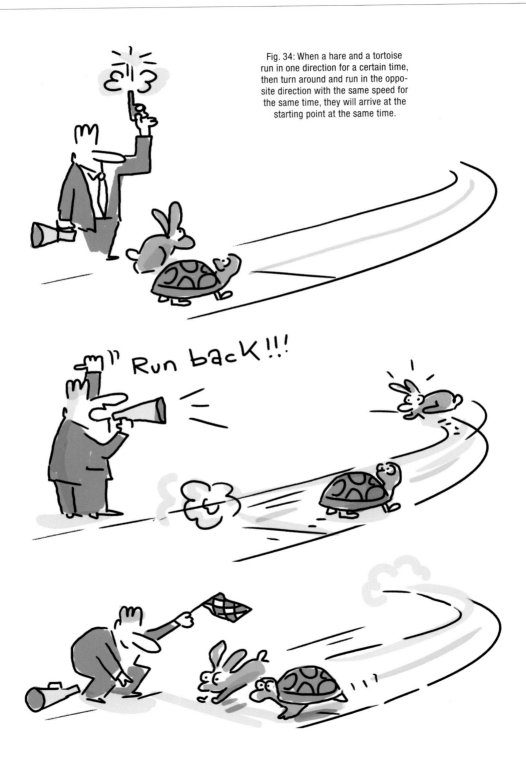

Fig. 34: When a hare and a tortoise run in one direction for a certain time, then turn around and run in the opposite direction with the same speed for the same time, they will arrive at the starting point at the same time.

To illustrate this: think about a race be-tween a tortoise and a hare starting at the same line (figure 34). After a certain time (TE/2), the hare is ahead of the tortoise. When you make the competitors run in the opposite direction for the same length of time, they will both be back at the starting line at exactly the same time (assuming, that they run at constant speed).

In our experiment, the **180° pulse** acts like a wall, from which the protons bounce back, like a mountain reflecting sound waves as echoes. This is why the resulting strong signal is also called an echo, or **spin echo**.

After we have our signal, our spin echo, the protons lose phase coherence again, the faster ones getting ahead, as we have seen.

We naturally can perform the experiment again with another 180° pulse, and another and another ...

If we now plot time vs. signal intensity, we get a curve like in figure 35.

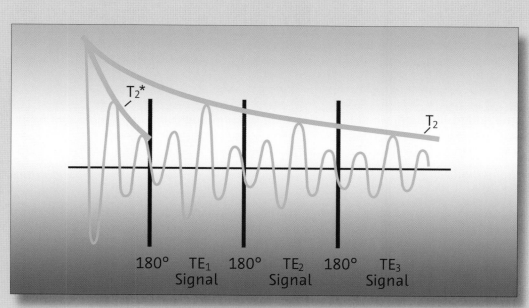

Fig. 35: The 180° pulse refocuses the dephasing protons, which results in a stronger signal, the spin echo after the time TE. The protons then dephase again and can be refocused anoth-er time by a 180° pulse, and so on. Thus it is possible to obtain more than one signal, more than one spin echo. The spin echoes, however, differ in intensity due to so-called T_2-effects. A curve connecting the spin echo intensities is the T_2-curve. If we did not use the 180° pulse, the signal intensity would decay much faster. A curve describing the signal intensity in that case is the **T_2^*-(T_2 star)** curve, which is described in a little more detail on page 52.

From this curve we can see that the spin echo, the resulting signal, decreases with time. Responsible for this is the fact that our 180° pulse only "neutralizes" effects that influence the protons in a constant manner, and these are the constant inhomogeneities of the external magnetic field.

Inconstant inhomogeneities from local magnetic fields inside the tissue cannot be "evened out", as they may influence some protons before the 180° pulse differently than after the 180° pulse. So some of the protons may still be behind or in front of the majority of the protons that will reach the starting line at the same time. So from echo to echo, the intensity of the signal goes down due to so-called T_2-effects. A curve connecting the spin echo intensities is the T_2-curve.

Maybe we should illustrate this by an example: imagine two buses full of people, e.g. after a soccer or football game. They are standing at a starting line (figure 36). With two microphones, you record the signal (e.g. the singing from the crowd) that is coming from each bus. The buses leave in the same direction.

Listening to the singing of the crowds, i.e. recording the signal, you may recognize that one signal disappears faster than the other.

This can have two different causes: The difference in signal intensities, the difference in singing, may be due to differences in inherent properties of the two groups (internal inhomogeneities); maybe in one bus, there are only the "party animals", who did not become tired as fast as the people in the other crowd.

Or . . . maybe one bus is driving faster than the other (loss of signal would thus be due to external influences, the external magnetic field inhomogeneities).

To figure out what is actually the reason for the signal disappearing, you can make the buses turn around after a certain time TE/2, and have them drive back with the

same speed also for the time TE/2. After 2 x TE/2 = TE, the buses will be back at the starting line. The signal intensity that you record with your microphone then depends only on inherent properties, i.e. how tired the crowds have become.

Let us have a look at our curve, when we plotted time vs. signal intensity sending in several 180° pulses (see figure 35). If you do not use a 180° pulse to neutralize constant external inhomogeneities, the protons will experience larger differences in magnetic field strength, when the RF pulse is switched off. Due to this, they will be out of phase faster, the transversal relaxation time will be shorter.

A curve describing the signal intensity in that case is the T_2^*- (T_2 star) curve. The star distinguishes this shorter transversal relaxation time from the T_2 after the 180° pulse, which we have already talked about.

The corresponding effects are named T_2^*-effects. These T_2^*-effects are important with the so-called fast imaging sequences; we will hear about them later.

In our example with the buses, this would mean that we just record the signals as the buses drive away. The signals vanish due to extrinsic (bus speed) and intrinsic (exhaustion of the passengers) properties under these circumstances (see figure 36).

The type of pulse sequence that we used in our experiment is called a **spin echo sequence**, consisting of a 90° pulse and a 180° pulse (causing the echo). This pulse sequence is very important in MR imaging, as it is the workhorse among the pulse sequences, which can be used for many things. It is important to realize that with a spin echo sequence, we cannot only produce T_2-, but also T_1- and proton density-weighted images. We will get to that a little later.

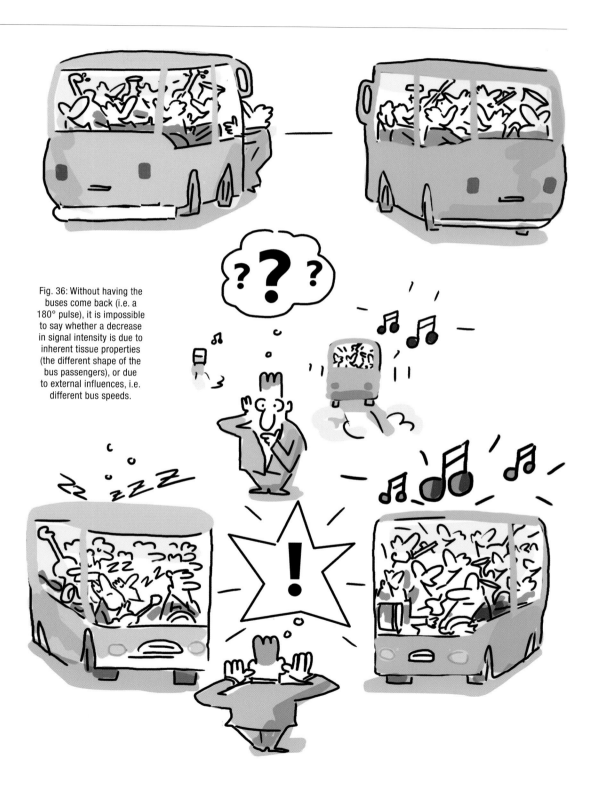

Fig. 36: Without having the buses come back (i.e. a 180° pulse), it is impossible to say whether a decrease in signal intensity is due to inherent tissue properties (the different shape of the bus passengers), or due to external influences, i.e. different bus speeds.

Let us first look at such a T_2-weighted sequence

What did we do? First, we sent in a 90° pulse, resulting in some transversal magnetization. Immediately after the 90° pulse, we have a maximum transversal magnetization. However, this transversal magnetization disappears, due to **T_2-effects**. How fast transversal magnetization disappears, can be seen from a **T_2-curve**; in figure 37, we have plotted T_2-curves for two different tissues, tissue A having a short T_2 (e.g. brain), tissue B having a long T_2 (water or CSF). The curves start at 0, which is the time immediately after the 90° pulse is switched off. When we wait for

a certain time TE/2 to send in the 180° pulse, transversal magnetization will have become smaller. After waiting another time TE/2 (that is TE after the 90° pulse is switched off), we will receive a signal, the spin echo.

The intensity of this echo is given by the T_2-curve at the time TE. This time between the 90° pulse and the spin echo is called **TE = time to echo**.

The time TE can be chosen by the operator. And as we can see from the T_2-curve, TE influences the resulting signal, and thus also the image: the shorter the time TE, the stronger the signal that we get from a tissue. To get the best, strong signal, it may seem reasonable to use a short TE, because with longer TEs, signal intensity decreases. With a short TE, however, there will be a problem (figure 37).

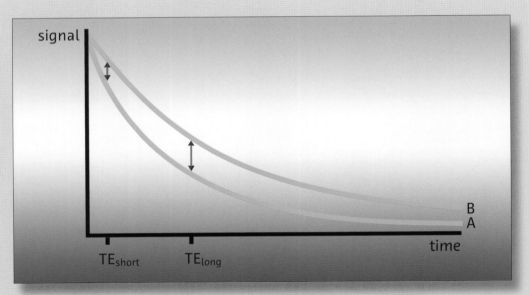

Fig. 37: T_2-curves for two tissues with different transversal relaxation times; tissue A has a shorter T_2 than tissue B, thus loses transversal magnetization faster. With a short TE (TE$_{short}$), the difference in signal intensity is less pronounced than after a longer TE (TE$_{long}$).

Let us have a look at two different tissues. Tissue B (water or CSF) has a longer T_2 than tissue A (brain).

Both T_2-curves in this example start at the same point. If we only wait a short TE, TE_{short}, the difference in signal intensity between tissue A and tissue B is very small, both tissues may hardly be distinguished, as there is hardly any contrast (which is the difference in signal intensity of tissues).

Consequence: with a short TE, differences in T_2 do not influence tissue contrast very much.

As both T_2-curves diverge with a longer TE, TE_{long}, the difference in T_2-curves, and thus the difference in signal intensity meaning **contrast**, is more pronounced in our example. So it might be reasonable to wait a very long TE; the resulting image should be very heavily T_2-weighted. But (and there is always a "but") if we wait longer, the total signal intensity becomes smaller and smaller. The **signal-to-noise ratio** becomes smaller, the image appears grainy.

An example to illustrate this signal-to-noise problem: when you receive a local radio station in your radio, this gives you a good signal, e.g. loud music and only little static noise.

When you drive out of town, the signal intensity of the radio station becomes weaker, and you will hear more static noise; and when you drive even further away, you may not be able to discern the music from the background noise. And this is the same for the MR signal: there is always some noise in the system, however, when the signal is strong, this does not matter much. However, the smaller the signal, the harder it is to differentiate it from the background noise.

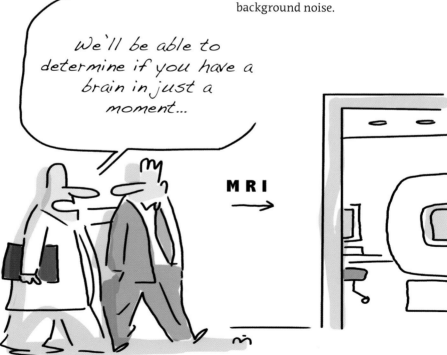

Let us review some facts

We have learned:
- The spin echo sequence consists of a 90° and a 180° pulse.
- After the 90° pulse, protons dephase due to external and internal magnetic field inhomogeneities.
- The 180° pulse rephases the dephasing protons (sometimes the term "spins" is used interchangeably for protons), and a stronger signal, the spin echo, results.
- The 180° pulse serves to "neutralize" the external magnetic field inhomogeneities.
- Signal decrease from one echo to the next, when using multiple 180° pulses, is due to internal T_2-effects.
- By choosing different TEs (different times after the 90° pulse), the signal can be T_2-weighted in varying degrees – with very short TEs, T_2-effects have not yet had time to really show up.
- With longer TEs, the signal intensity difference between tissues will depend very much on their T_2s, their transversal relaxation time.
- With very long TEs, there should be even more T_2-weighting, however, signal intensity as such would be so small that at best it can just barely be distinguished from the background noise.

By the way: what is a short, what is a long TR or TE?

A short **TR** is one that is about as short as the smallest/shortest T_1 that we are interested in (remember: T_1 was a time constant, not a time that it takes for a tissue to regain its longitudinal magnetization!). A long TR is about 3 times as long as a short TR. A TR of less than 500 msec is considered to be short, a TR of more than 1,500 msec to be long (just to give you a rough idea). A short TE is one that is as short as possible, a long TE also is more than 3 times as long.

A TE of less than 20 msec is considered to be short, a TE more than 80 msec to be long.

The pattern of a spin echo sequence

Let us go back to our spin echo pulse sequence.

This sequence can be illustrated schematically as in figure 38: 90° pulse – wait TE/2 – 180° pulse – wait TE/2 – record signal. For certain different reasons, such a pulse sequence is repeated two or more times. The time to repeat a pulse sequence was TR, time to repeat. So what we get is the following scheme:

1. 90° pulse – TE/2 – 180° pulse – TE/2 – recording signal at TE.
After TR (time from the beginning of one 90° pulse to the next 90° pulse) follows another pulse cycle and signal measurement:

2. 90° pulse – TE/2 – 180° pulse – TE/2 – recording signal at TE.

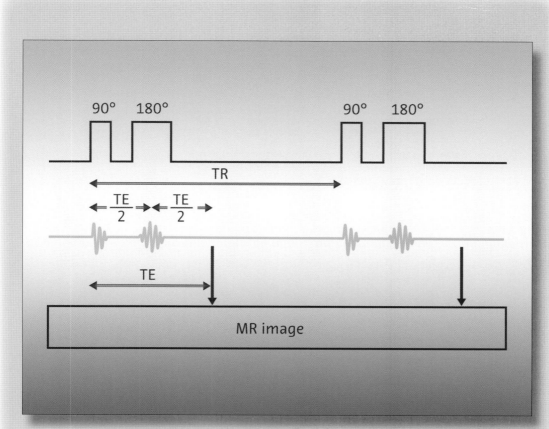

Fig. 38: Schematic illustration of a spin echo pulse sequence.

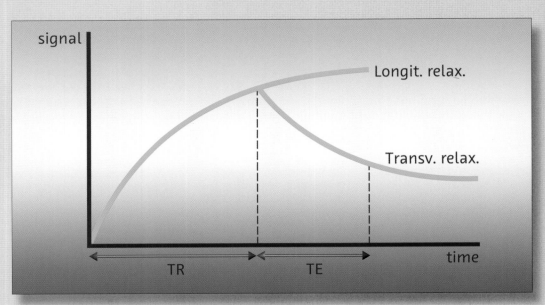

Fig. 39: It is possible to determine signal intensity for a tissue using a **spin echo sequence** by combining the T_1- and the T_2-curve for that tissue. The longitudinal magnetization after the time TR is equal to the amount of transversal magnetization we start out with, as it is "tilted" 90 degrees. This transversal magnetization immediately starts to disappear by a rate which is determined by the transversal relaxation time, and thus by the T_2-curve. The signal intensity of the tissue after a time TE can then be inferred from the T_2-curve at this time TE (which starts after TR!).

TR and TE

To figure out how much signal you get from a certain tissue with certain parameters of a **spin echo sequence**, you actually have to do no more than combine its T_1- and T_2-curves, as it is illustrated in figure 39. Here we have the T_1- and T_2-curve of a certain tissue. T_1 represents the longitudinal relaxation and T_2 represents the transversal relaxation. Which parameter determined the amount of **longitudinal magnetization**? That was TR. To see

how much longitudinal magnetization will be tilted 90° to the side (and thus to figure out, with how much transversal magnetization we start out with), we just look at the intensity of the longitudinal magnetization at the time **TR**.

The **longitudinal magnetization** at this point, "tilted" in the transversal plane, is the starting point from which transversal magnetization decays. So we just attach the **T_2-curve** at this point.

How much signal we get with a spin echo sequence to construct the image,

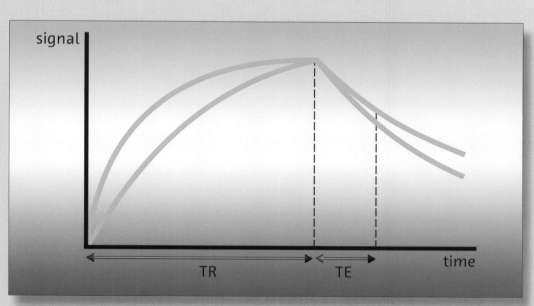

Fig. 40: By combining T_1- and T_2-curves, signal intensity of certain tissues can be determined for a pulse sequence using TR and TE as illustrated, and as explained in figure 39. What happens, when we choose a long TR, as illustrated? With a long TR, differences in T_1, in longitudinal magnetization time are not very important any more, as all tissues have regained their full longitudinal magnetization. When we only wait a very short TE, then differences in signal intensity due to differences in T_2 have not yet had time to become pronounced. The resulting image is thus neither T_1- nor T_2-weighted, but mostly determined by the proton density of the tissues (for this, ideally TE should be zero).

also depends on TE, the time that we wait after the 90° pulse. So we now only have to look for the signal intensity at the time TE on the **T_2-curve**.

What image do we get, when we choose a long TR and a short TE?

This is illustrated in figure 40. Here are the T_1- and T_2-curves for two different tissues.

As we heard earlier, with a very long TR, all tissues will have totally recovered their longitudinal magnetization; differences in T_1 of the tissues examined will not influence the signal,

as enough time has passed by to allow even tissues with a long T_1 to relax totally. So when we choose a long TR, as we just said, then differences in T_1 do not really matter.

When we also use a short TE, differences in signal intensity due to differences in T_2 have not had enough time to become pronounced yet.

The signal that we get, is thus neither T_1- nor T_2-weighted, but mainly influenced by differences in **proton** or **spin density**.

The more protons, the more signal, if you look at it simply (figure 40).

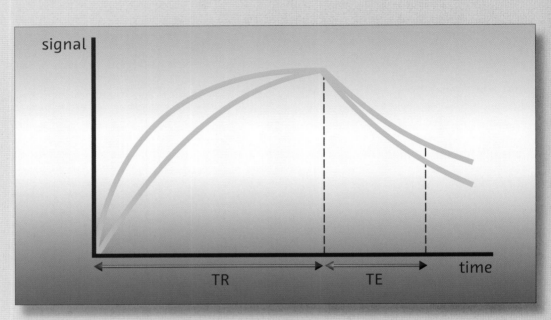

Fig. 41: When we wait a long TR and a long TE, differences in T_2 have had time enough to become pronounced, the resulting picture is T_2-weighted.

And what happens when we use a long TR and a long TE?

With a long TR, there are no prevailing differences in T_1. With the long TE, however, differences in T_2 become pronounced. Thus the resulting image is T_2-weighted (figure 41).

What if we use a shorter TR and a short TE?

With a short TR, tissues have not re-covered their longitudinal magnetization, thus differences in T_1 (which determines how fast longitudinal magnetization is regained) will show up in form of signal intensity differences (figure 42).

When TE is short, differences in T_2 cannot really manifest themselves, so the resulting image is still T_1-weighted (there is a lower limit for TE, because it takes some time for the 180°

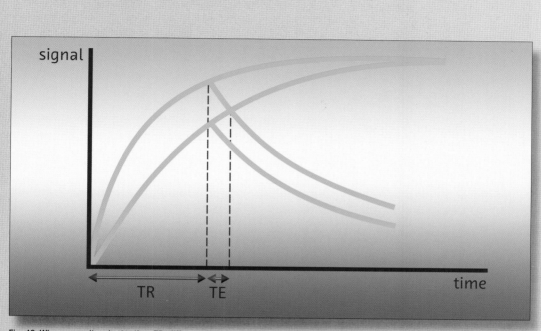

Fig. 42: When we wait a shorter time TR, differences in T_1 influence tissue contrast to a larger extent, the picture is T_1-weighted, especially when we also wait a short TE (when signal differences due to differing T_2s have not had time to become pronounced).

pulse to be "produced", sent in and to properly take effect).

What if we use a very short TR and a very long TE?

This is only a theoretical question. Why?

With a very short TR, there will only be very little longitudinal magnetization which is "tilted". And with a long TE, we even allow the small amount of transversal magnetization resulting to disappear to a large extent. The resulting signal will be so small, of so little intensity that it cannot be used to make a reasonable image.

If you have not been concentrating

for the last few minutes, you are probably thinking about giving up right now. How to remember this – even if you do not understand all of it (which hopefully is not the case)?

Try looking at figure 43. What can you see? A man with short TRousers. And considering the weather conditions, this makes only one person in the picture happy.

This should remind you that a short TR (TRousers) gives a T_1-weighted image (only 1 is happy).

And what do you see in figure 44? The same couple is having tea. Now, having tea which is usually served hot, always takes a long time. And in the illustration the long TEa makes two people happy. This should remind you that a long TE gives a T_2-weighted image.

Fig. 43: What to choose for a T_1-weighted image?

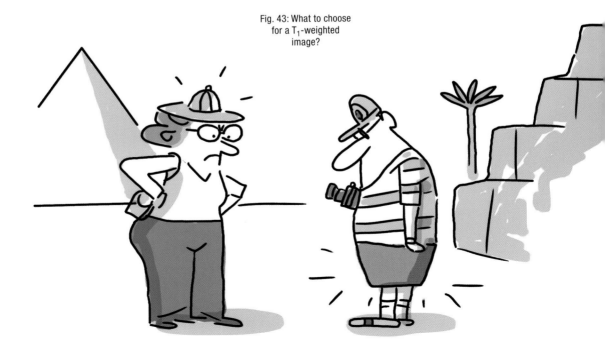

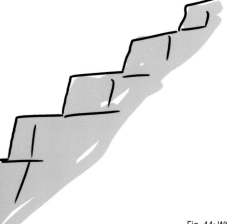

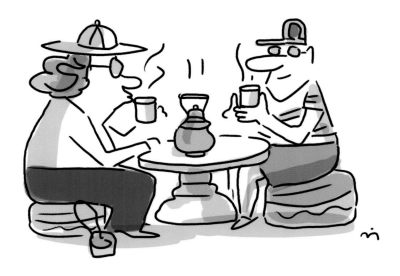

Fig. 44: What to choose
for a T_2-weighted
image?

Fig. 45: T$_1$- (A), proton (spin) density- (B), and T$_2$-weighted (C) images of the same patient. The CSF is black on the T$_1$-weighted image. However, it has the strongest signal in the T$_2$-weighted image. On the spin-density image, it is of intermediate signal intensity.

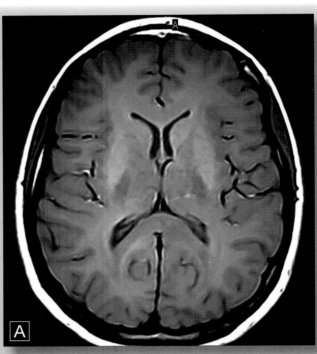

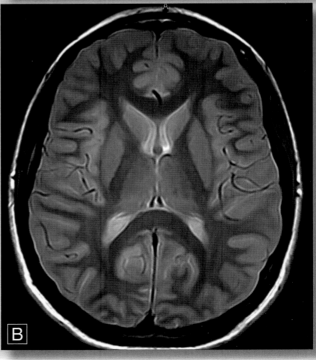

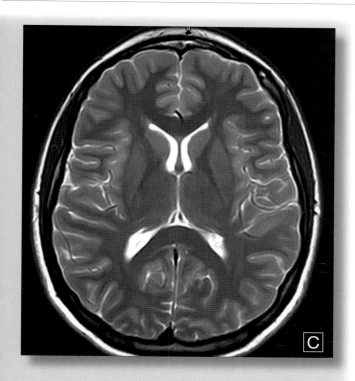

Some practical hints to image interpretation

How can we tell from an image, whether it is a T_1- or a T_2-weighted image, when imaging was done with a normal pulse sequence, not one of the fast sequences (which we will hear about a little later)?

As a rule of thumb: if you see white fluid, e.g. CSF or urine, you are dealing with a T_2-weighted image. If the fluid is darker than the solids, we have a T_1- or a proton-density image.

Look at the scan (figure 45): CSF is dark, the grey matter is darker (greyer) than the white matter; this is a typical **T_1-weighted image**.

In (B), CSF is still dark, even though its signal intensity is slightly higher than in the T_1-weighted image; contrast between the grey and white matter is becoming reversed. This is a proton or spin density-weighted image, and as the grey matter has a higher water content, i.e. contains more protons, its signal intensity is higher than that of the white substance.

In (C), CSF has a higher signal intensity than grey and white matter, the image is **T_2-weighted**.

These are rules of thumb only. Actually, to be really sure, you would have to look at two images taken with different imaging parameters. Why?

Look at figure 46. You can see that in this example the T_2-curves start at different "heights", and cross each other.

They do not have to run parallel, as we depicted them in the previous illustration, which was only done for didactic reasons, as it is easier to understand at the beginning.

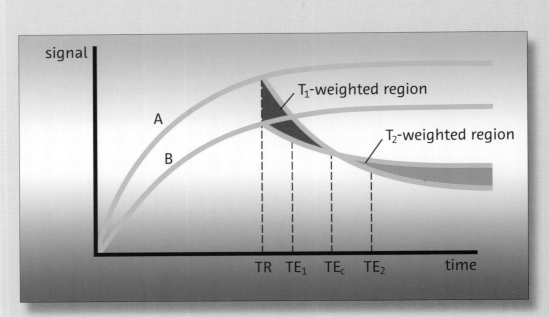

Fig. 46: T_2-curves of different tissues can intersect. The signal intensity of the tissues is reversed choosing a TE beyond the crossing point (TE_C): before this crossing point (e.g. at TE_1), tissue A has a higher signal intensity than tissue B. This means that image contrast is still determined by differences in T_1: the tissue A with the shorter T_1 has the stronger signal intensity. At TE_C, both tissues have the same signal intensity, and thus cannot be differentiated. After this crossing point (e.g. at TE_2), the relative signal intensities are reversed, and tissue B has the stronger signal.

The fact that the curves intersect is very important:
● With a TE before the crossing point (TE_1), tissue A will have a higher signal intensity.
● With a TE right at that point (TE_C), we cannot distinguish the tissues at all, as they have the same signal intensity.

Thus, you might be unlucky, and choose a pulse sequence with just those imaging parameters that do not allow tissue differentiation (which is the reason for performing two different examinations with different T_1- and T_2-weightings).

● With a TE beyond the crossing point (TE_2), tissue A will have a lower signal than tissue B.
● Before this crossing point (which you do not know, looking at an image normally), the relative signal intensities are still governed by differences in T_1.

The tissue with the shorter T_1 (or the higher proton density, if we have a long TR) still has the higher signal intensity.

Only with longer TEs does the T_2-weighting come up. Think about that for a moment!

How does flow influence the signal?

Now we have already heard about many parameters that influence the MR image, T_1, T_2, proton density, pulse sequences, TR and TE – but there are more, e.g. contrast media, and flow.

The fact that **flow** influences the MR signal has been known for a long time. The first experiments on this subject were carried out more than forty years ago. Interestingly, this phenomenon was used to measure flow in the fuel pipes of satellite rockets, without having to put any obstruction into the flow lines.

The subject of how flow influences the MR signal is rather complex and difficult, but let us at least get some idea about it.

In figure 47, we have a body section through which a vessel is crossing.

When we send in our first 90° pulse, all the protons in the cross section are influenced by the radio wave. After we turn the RF pulse off, we "listen" into the section and record a signal.

At this time, all the original blood in our vessel may have left the slice being examined. So there is no signal coming out of the vessel; it appears black in the image. This phenomenon is called **flow-void** phenomenon.

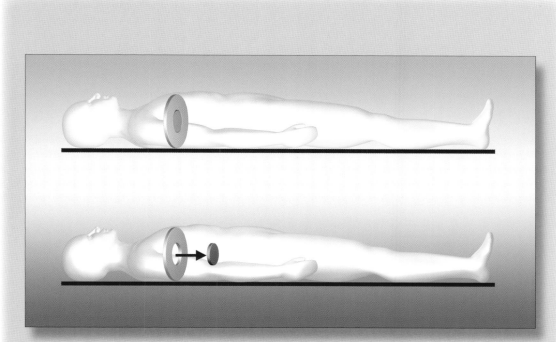

Fig. 47: Flow effects are responsible for the black appearance of flowing blood, the signal void in blood vessels.

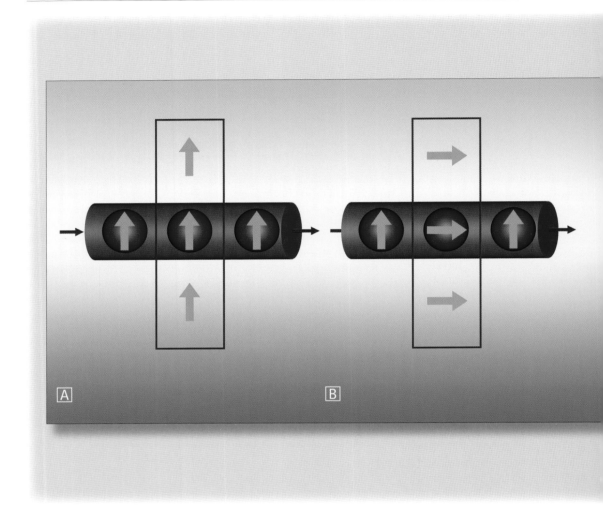

This is not the only way in which flow may influence the image, there may be all kinds of things, e.g. also flow-related enhancement.

Illustration 48 shows a blood vessel going through a slice which is being examined. (A) represents the situation before the 90° pulse and (B) immediately after the pulse, longitudinal magnetization is "tilted" 90°.

If we wait some more time, before we send in a second 90° pulse, like in (C), protons will have undergone some relaxation, and there is some longitudinal magnetization again, as shown by the arrows pointing back up. The protons in the blood vessel, however, have left the slice and been replaced by protons that still have all of their longitudinal magnetization.

If we send in a second 90° pulse now, there will be more signal coming from the vessel than from its surroundings, because there is more longitudinal magnetization at this

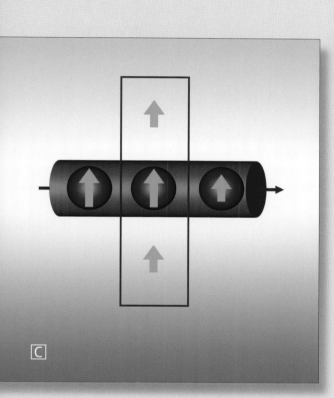

Fig. 48: Flow can have differing effects on signal intensity, and can also cause flow-related enhancement, which is explained in detail in the text.

time. The whole subject of signal strength and flow effects is actually much more complicated.

For example, when you do multi-slice imaging, i.e. taking images of more than one slice at the same time (see page 83), the signal also depends on the direction of the **flow**. In addition, it differs over the cross section of a vessel, depending on the flow profile, and whether there is laminar or turbulent flow. If you want to know more about this, you should look it up in one of the comprehensive standard text books.

They will also give you more information on MRI angiography.

In this technique, the fact that flow influences the MRI signal is used positively by displaying the moving protons.

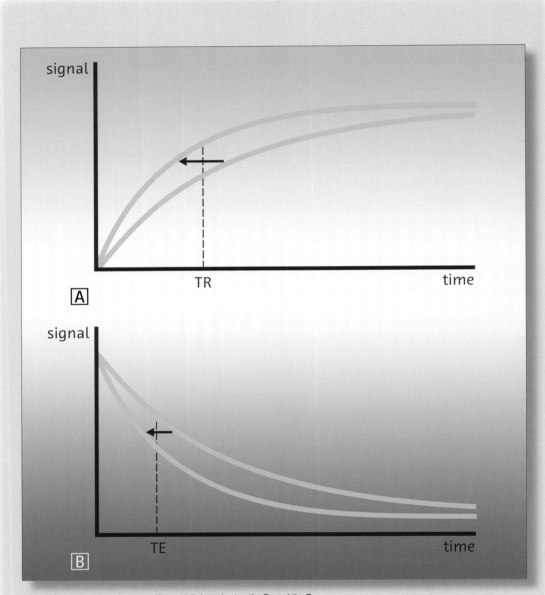

Fig. 49: Paramagnetic substances like gadolinium shorten the T_1 and the T_2 of their surroundings. The respective T_1- (fig. 49A) and T_2-curves (fig. 49B) are shifted towards the left. In effect, this means that for a certain TR there is more, for a certain TE, however, there is less signal.

What about MR contrast media?

Certain so-called **paramagnetic substances** have small local magnetic fields, which cause a shortening of the relaxation times of the protons in their neighborhood. This effect is named proton **relaxation enhancement**.

The body contains such paramagnetic substances under normal circumstances. Examples are degradation products of **hemoglobin**, e.g. **deoxyglobin** and **methemoglobin**, which are found in hematomas, or also molecular oxygen.

Gadolinium (Gd), a paramagnetic substance, is used in MR contrast media.

Chemically, Gadolinium is a rare earth metal, which, however, is toxic in its free state. Because of this it is bound to "some other chemical" in a certain way called chelation, which solves the problem of toxicity.

The Gd-containing **contrast media** have an effect on both the signal intensity of T_1- and T_2-weighted images, as they shorten the T_1 and the T_2 of their surroundings (figure 49), meaning that the respective curves are shifted towards the left.

In effect, for a given **TR**, there is more signal, for a given **TE**, there is less signal.

Now don't move for the next thirty minutes. If you really have to, you may breathe.

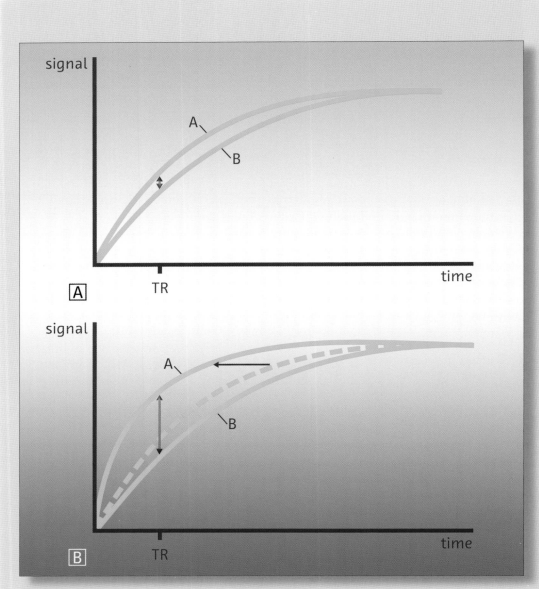

Fig. 50: In (A), the T_1-curves for tissue A and B are very close to each other, resulting in only a small difference in signal intensity between the tissues at TR. In (B), the T_1-curve of tissue A is shifted to the left, as contrast agent entered tissue A but not tissue B. At the same time TR, there now is a much greater difference in signal intensity, i.e. tissue contrast.

In figure 50, the signal intensity for two tissues, A and B, is illustrated. The i.v. administered Gd **contrast medium** enters tissue A, but not tissue B.

The T_1 of tissue A becomes shorter and the **T_1-curve** is shifted to the left.

The result is that the signal from tissue A at time TR is stronger than it was before, and the two tissues can be better differentiated, because there is better contrast.

What happens, when we perform a T_2-weighted examination after contrast medium application, we have seen in figure 49: the **T_2-curve** is shifted to the left, reducing the signal coming at a given TE.

As loss of signal is often more difficult to appreciate than a signal enhancement, T_1-weighted images are the predominant imaging technique used after contrast medium injection. As the **contrast media** are not distributed evenly throughout the body, signals from different tissues will be influenced differently. Vascularized tumor tissues are enhanced, for example. This may, for example, help with differentiation between tumor tissue and surrounding edema, which might otherwise be indistinguishable.

It is also important that the Gd compounds do not go through the intact, but only through the disrupted **blood-brain barrier**.

In general, it has been shown that the use of contrast media increases lesion detection and diagnostic accuracy of MRI in very many cases.

What magnetic field are you hanging around in?

Ready for a review?

 As we know by now, many parameters, e.g. T_1, T_2, proton density, pulse sequence parameters, influence the appearance of tissues in an MR image.

● With a short TR, we get a T_1-weighted image.

● With long TE, the image is T_2-weighted.

● Flow effects can be variable, and cover the spectrum from signal loss to signal enhancement.

● Paramagnetic substances, e.g. contrast media, shorten T_1 and T_2 of the surrounding protons. This results in a signal increase in T_1-weighted images and a signal decrease in T_2-weighted images.

● T_1-weighted imaging is the preferred technique after contrast medium injection.

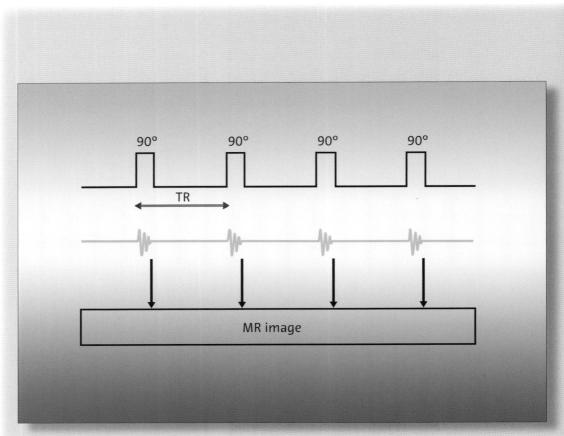

Fig. 51: Schematic illustration of the partial saturation/saturation recovery sequence.

Partial saturation/ saturation recovery sequence

We already heard about the term **pulse sequence**. Many different pulse sequences have been developed, and we should be familiar with their basic

concepts. So let us take a look at them. Pulse sequences that use 90° pulses only, are the **saturation recovery pulse sequence** and the **partial saturation sequence** (figure 51) (which we have already discussed, but we did not give them a name).

Basically, the sequences are the same: they consist of two 90° pulses. The dif-

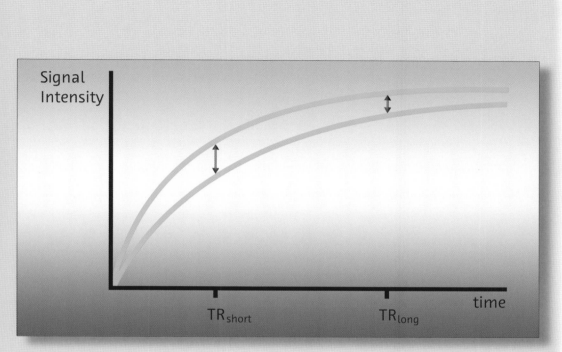

Fig. 52: Signal intensity of tissues having a different T_1 depending on the choice of TR: With a long TR, the saturation recovery sequence, image contrast is determined mainly by proton (spin) density. With a shorter TR, the partial saturation sequence, the resulting image is T_1-weighted.

ference is in the time interval between pulses, the TR (see page 45).

You can see the effect in figure 52 with the T_1-curves (going uphill!) of two different tissues. If we send in the second pulse after a long time, TR_{long}, both tissues will have regained longitudinal magnetization. With a TR_{long}, with the saturation recovery sequence (the protons have relaxed, are saturated), the signal is influenced by the proton density (Do you recall the stories with the short trousers and the long teas?). With a TR_{short}, with the partial saturation (protons have not relaxed), the T_1 becomes important for the signal intensity, so we get T_1-weighted images (figure 52).

Inversion recovery sequence

In contrast to the spin echo sequence that we have mentioned before (see page 57), the inversion recovery sequence uses first a 180° pulse which is then followed by a 90° pulse (figure 53).

What happens?

The 180° pulse turns the **longitudinal magnetization** in the opposite direction (all protons that were responsible

for the net magnetic moment pointing up, now point down).

This is illustrated in figure 54 for two tissues with different T_1. The tissue with the faster longitudinal relaxation, i.e. the shorter T_1, is in the bottom row.

If we do not do anything else, the longitudinal magnetization will slowly go back up, like a ball that is thrown into water. To get a measurable signal, however, we need some transversal magnetization. And for this, we use

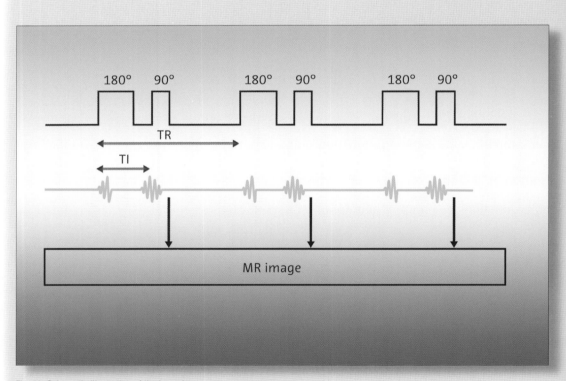

Fig. 53: Schematic illustration of the inversion recovery sequence.

the 90° pulse. The 90° pulse "tilts" the magnetization into the transversal (x-y-) plane, so it can be measured/received.

The signal that we get depends on the time between the 180°- and the 90° pulse, the time after the inversion by the 180° pulse; this time is thus called **TI = inversion time**.

The signal intensity in an **inversion recovery** image is dependent on T_1, which determines how fast the longitudinal magnetization goes back to its original value. So we get a T_1-weighted image – which is even more T_1-weighted than partial saturation recovery images.

Interestingly, when the 90° pulse is sent in when the longitudinal magnetization goes from negative to positive, i.e. is zero, the tissue does not give a signal! This may be useful when we do not want a tissue to show up in the image, e.g. when we want to suppress the fat signal – but let us not go into too much detail here.

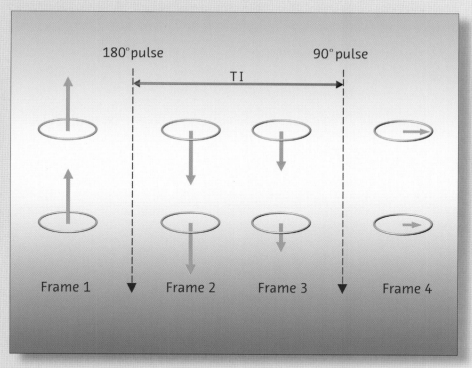

Fig. 54: The inversion recovery sequence uses a 180° pulse which inverts the longitudinal magnetization, followed by a 90° pulse after the time TI. The 90° pulse "tilts" the magnetization into the transversal (x-y-) plane, so it can be measured/received. The tissue in the bottom row goes back to its original longitudinal magnetization faster, thus has the shorter T_1. For the time TI which is illustrated, this results in less transversal magnetization after the 90° pulse.

Spin echo sequence

We have talked about the spin echo sequence in detail already.

It is composed of two pulses: a 90°- and a 180° pulse (figure 55).

You should be able to recall what happens by now: The 90° pulse establishes transversal magnetization, which immediately starts to decrease because the protons dephase. Some time (TE/2) after the 90° pulse, we send in a 180° pulse, which rephases the protons.

After the time **TE**, we get a strong signal, the **spin echo**. As we have heard, we can produce not only one, but several echoes using more than one 180° pulse.

The disadvantage is, however that the signal becomes weaker and weaker.

What were the imaging parameters that influenced the MR signal in the spin echo sequences?

These were: **TE** = the time between the 90° pulse and the echo and **TR** = the time between two pulse sequences, i.e. from one 90° pulse to the next.

What did the TE and the TR do?

They determined how the resulting image was weighted: TE was responsible for the T_2-weighting, TR for the T_1-weighting.

If you cannot remember this or still are feeling unsure, please go back to pages 48 – 63 again.

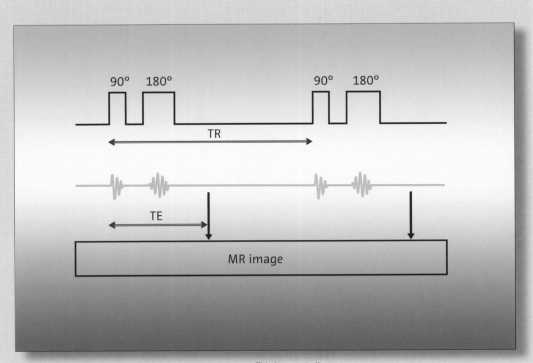

Fig. 55: Schematic illustration of a spin echo pulse sequence. This is repeatedly illustrated, as the spin echo sequence is so important.

What about those fast imaging sequences?

Normal imaging sequences take quite some time, during which it may be difficult for the patient to lay completely still. In addition, there is always some unavoidable motion, like respiration and heart beat. All these movements unfortunately decrease image quality.

To help with these problems, **fast pulse sequences** were developed, which take less time. Most of these have strange names such as FLASH (Fast – Low – Angle – Shot), or GRASS (Gradient – Recalled – Acquisition – at Steady – State). These sequences are very important nowadays in daily practice.

As you may already have noticed, the TR is the most time consuming parameter of an imaging sequence (see also pages 57 and 83). It makes sense to shorten TR if we want to make imaging faster. And this is done in the fast imaging sequences.

But with a decreasing TR, there are some problems:
● Firstly, with a spin echo sequence we used a 180° pulse to refocus the dephasing spins. Unfortunately, we cannot use a 180° pulse for this purpose, when we do imaging with a very short TR: it requires some time to "produce" and to deliver a 180° pulse, and with a very short TR, there will not be enough time for that between the 90° pulses.
● Secondly, with decreasing TR, longitudinal magnetization will have recovered less and less between pulses (see pages 58-61), as we have already seen; so there is only very little longitudinal magnetization to be tilted by the next pulse, yielding very little signal.

These problems are solved as follows:
● We use a different way to refocus the dephasing spins: instead of a 180° pulse, we apply a **magnetic field gradient**. This means that an uneven magnetic field, a gradient field, is added/superimposed on the existing magnetic field.

The magnetic field gradient is switched on for a short time. This results in even larger magnetic field inhomogeneities in the examined slice. (The magnetic field inhomogeneities that already exist at that time are due to inhomogeneities of the external magnetic field, and the internal magnetic field inhomogeneities inside of the tissues, which we talked about earlier – if you do not remember this, go back to page 27 for a short recap).

Due to these larger magnetic field inhomogeneities, **transversal magnetization**, and thus the signal, disappears faster (protons dephase faster!). Then the magnetic gradient is switched off, and after a short time turned back on with the same strength, but in the opposite direction.

The faster moving protons now become the ones that move slowly, and vice versa (similar to what happens after a 180° pulse).

This results in some rephasing, and thus the signal increases again to a certain maximum, which is called a **gradient echo**. After this echo, the signal decreases again.

What to do about the second problem, the small amount of longitudinal magnetization with a short TR? The 90° pulse, e.g. in a spin echo sequence, abolishes longitudinal magnetization; longitudinal magnetization, however, starts to recover immediately after the 90° pulse, depending on the T_1 of the tissue examined (if you have forgotten, see page 38). The trick with the fast imaging sequences is not to use a 90° pulse, but pulses that cause smaller **"flip angles"** (mostly in the range of 10°-35°).

With these flip angles smaller than 90 degrees, **longitudinal magnetization** is not totally abolished. Instead, there is always a substantial amount of longitudinal magnetization left, which can be "tilted" by the next pulse; this gives a reasonable signal even if the next pulse comes in after a very short TR.

As we have heard, a 180° pulse normally "neutralizes" the effects of external magnetic field inhomogeneities. The decay of transversal magnetization is then due to so-called T_2**-effects** (see figure 35).

When we do not use such a 180° pulse, the protons experience larger magnetic field inhomogeneities and get out of phase faster. Signal intensity decays faster, and in this case is due to so-called T_2***-effects** (pronounced: T_2 star-effects), which has already been illustrated in figure 35.

Besides these T_2*-effects, other factors, e.g. the **flip angle**, influence signal intensity in the fast imaging sequences, which are also called **gradient echo sequences** for obvious reasons.

Here are some guidelines about gradient echo imaging:

● Larger flip angles produce more T_1-weighting.
● Longer TEs produce more T_2*-weighting.
● With fast scans, intense signals often come out of the vessels.

We save imaging time because
– with small flip angles we only need an **RF pulse** of short duration;

– we do not use a 180° refocusing pulse (which takes time to be generated and to take effect);
– we do not have to wait long TRs for enough longitudinal magnetization to reappear, as with small flip angles there is always a reasonable amount of longitudinal magnetization left after the initial pulse.

With these fast scans, it is possible to do imaging in a second or even less.

Well, time to repeat and take a break.

Partial saturation and saturation recovery sequences use 90° pulses. TR is relatively short with partial saturation and relatively long with saturation recovery.

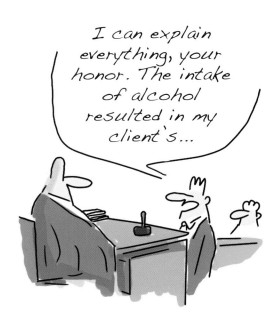

I can explain everything, your honor. The intake of alcohol resulted in my client's...

While saturation recovery yields proton (spin) density images, the images are T_1-weighted with partial saturation.

● A spin echo sequence has a 90° pulse, which is followed by one – or more – 180° pulses, to rephase the dephasing protons resulting in one – or more – spin echoes. This sequence can give proton density-weighted, T_1-weighted, or T_2-weighted images. This is determined by the imaging parameters which are chosen (TR, TE).

● In the inversion recovery sequence, a 180° pulse is followed by a 90° pulse, resulting in T_1-weighted images.

● Fast imaging sequences use flip angles that are smaller than 90°, and so-called gradient echoes. Image weighting is also determined by the specific type of sequence and the imaging parameters chosen.

About imaging time

As we have just seen, fast imaging sequences decrease **imaging time**.

Is there any other way to decrease this time? What does actually determine the **imaging time**?

For MR imaging with normal pulse sequences, this can be easily calculated; the **acquisition time (a.t.)** is:

a.t. = TR x N x N_{ex}

This looks a little complicated but it isn't really. Let us start at the back. N_{ex} is the number of excitations. What does that mean?

For certain reasons, it is necessary to use not only one signal measurement, but to repeat the measurement several times. As the MR signal coming out of the patient is very weak, it may be good to add up signals from several measurements, to take several "**averages**", to get a good quality image.

Actually, what you get is an image with a better signal-to-noise ratio.

Naturally, imaging time increases with every additional measurement.

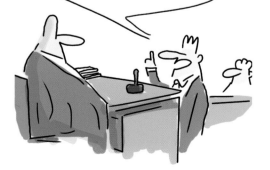

...increased spin, which in turn initiated a magnetization...

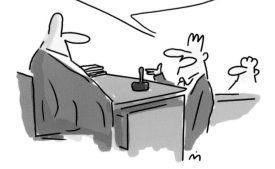

...that caused the coins in the till to become magically attracted to him.

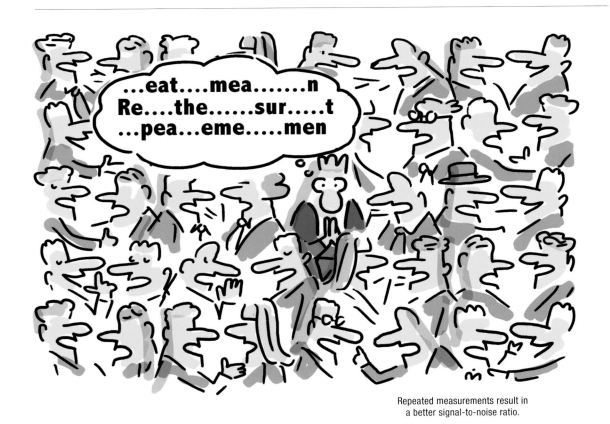

Repeated measurements result in a better signal-to-noise ratio.

To illustrate this: Just imagine that you are sitting in a large audience, where people are making a lot of noise. Someone sitting next to you whispers something in your ear, but you cannot really understand him, because there is so much background noise. What you will probably do, is ask him to repeat what he said once or several times. You mentally add up the information which you receive each time. As this signal is always the same, it will increase by adding it up. The **background noise**, however, is not always the same.

Instead, it is random and fluctuates and does not add up the way the signal does. So altogether you will have a better **signal-to-noise ratio** (which you would also have if the person spoke louder). Back to our formula: What is "N"? As you know from other imaging methods (or your PC), pictures are made of **picture elements**, which all together make up the image matrix, e.g. a 1,024 x 768 matrix has 768 rows of 1,024 picture elements (**pixels**).

In our equation, N is the number of rows in a **matrix**, like rows in a letter.

The more rows you have, the more time it takes for the image.

Just think about this as if you were writing a letter: if you have paper with 5 rows on a page, you will finish a page faster than if you have 25 rows to write. However, you have more content, more detail on a page/picture, when you work with more rows.

And why does TR influence acquisition time?

If you choose a long time TR to repeat your pulse sequence, to perform additional signal measurements, imaging takes longer than with a short TR. However, there is a trick that can shorten imaging time a bit.

While we are waiting to repeat our imaging sequence in one slice, i.e. while we wait for TR to go by (slice A in figure 56), we might as well make measurements in one or more different slices (slices B, C and D in figure 56).

The longer the TR, the more slices we can excite in the meantime.

So by just adding a little extra time, we will examine many slices instead of one, and imaging time per slice decreases substantially.

We perform so-called **multislice imaging**. Another way to possibly reduce TR, and thus imaging time, is the use of a **contrast medium**.

And when T_1 is shorter, the TR can also be shorter, without a loss in signal intensity of the tissue in question (see figure 49).

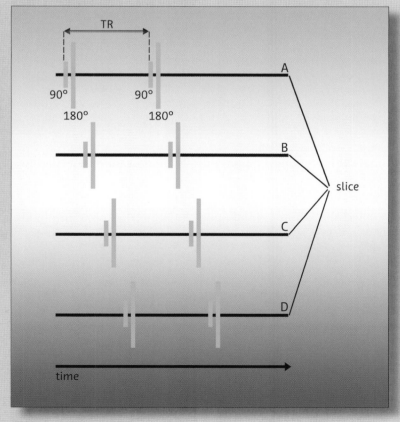

Fig. 56: Multislice imaging: while we wait for the time TR to pass by for another signal measurement in slice A, we perform signal measurements in additional slices. So during time TR, we actually recorded signals for more than one slice.

Let us review important factors that influence signal intensity in MR.

These are:
- proton density (page 45)
- T_1 (page 24)
- T_2 (page 28)
- flow (page 67)
- the pulse sequence (page 74-80)
- TR (page 45)
- TE (page 54)
- TI (page 77)
- flip angle (page 80)
- use of contrast medium (page 71)

If you are not sure about any of these, go back to the corresponding page.

If you feel familiar with these facts, continue with the next section, and learn about some important things in MR imaging that we have not talked about yet.

How can we select a slice which we want to examine?

When we put a patient into an MR scanner, he or she is in a rather homogeneous magnetic field.

So all the protons in the whole body have the same **Larmor frequency**, and will be excited/disturbed by the same RF pulse. To examine a specific slice only, a second magnetic field is superimposed on the external field, which has different strengths in varying locations. The magnetic field is therefore stronger or weaker in some places than in others (figure 57).

This additional field is called a **gradient field**, and is produced by the so-called **gradient coils**. This gradient field modifies the strength of the original magnetic field.

In figure 57, magnetic field strength increases for different cross sections from the feet towards the head.

Consequently, the protons in the different slices experience different magnetic fields, and thus have different precession frequencies.

So the RF pulses which disturb the protons in the different slices, must have different frequencies as well – otherwise there would be no resonance.

As gradient fields can be superimposed in any direction, it is possible to define not only transversal slices, but all kinds of different imaging planes without moving the patient. The gradient field that enables us to examine a specific slice, is also called **slice selecting gradient**.

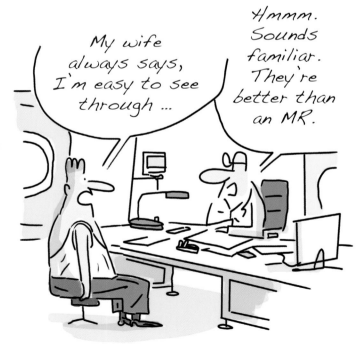

My wife always says, I'm easy to see through ...

Hmmm. Sounds familiar. They're better than an MR.

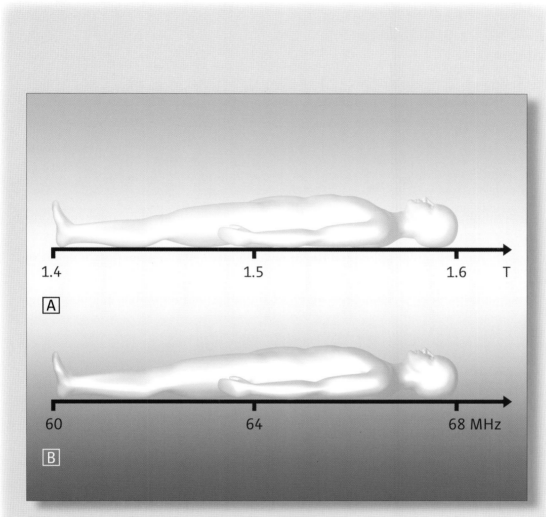

Fig. 57: Magnetic gradient fields are superimposed on the field of the MR magnet, so that different cross sections of the body experience magnetic fields of differing strength. In the illustration, the resulting magnetic field strength is increasing from 1.4 Tesla at the feet to 1.6 Tesla at the head. As magnetic field strength and precessing/resonant frequency are directly correlated (Larmor equation), the resonant frequency at the feet is about 60 MHz, while it is about 68 MHz at the top of the head in our example. By selecting a certain RF pulse frequency, we determine the location of the slice which we examine.

How can we determine or select a certain slice thickness?

We can select a different **slice thickness** in two ways (figure 58):

One solution is to send in not only one specific frequency (which is not done in practice), but an RF pulse that has a range of frequencies, which is often referred to as **bandwidth**; the wider the range of frequencies, the wider the bandwidth, the thicker the slice in which protons will be excited. This is illustrated in figure 58.

If we use an **RF pulse** with frequencies from 64 to 65 MHz, we will get the thickness of slice 1 (figure 58A). If, however, we only use frequencies from 64 to 64.5 MHz, the protons in the thinner slice 2, will show resonance (figure 58B).

There is another way to select a different slice thickness:

In our example, we used a gradient field that "produced" precessing or resonant frequencies starting at 60 MHz at the feet, up to 68 MHz at the top of the head. If we, however, have a steeper gradient field, i.e. one that has more difference in field strength over a specific distance, the precession frequencies will also vary to a larger degree, let us say from 56 MHz to 72 MHz.

If we now use an RF pulse of the same bandwidth as in A, containing frequencies between 64 and 65 MHz, the slice thickness in our example C with the steeper gradient field is, however, smaller than in our example A with the more shallow gradient field.

So using the same range of radio frequencies, the same bandwidth as it is called, slice thickness can be modified by the slope of the gradient field.

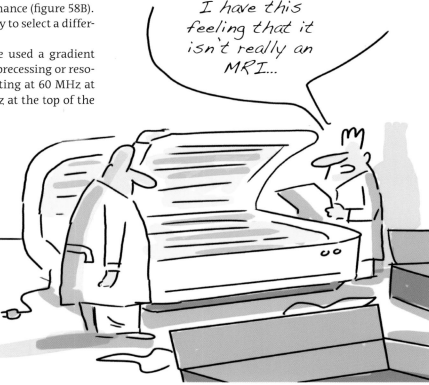

I have this feeling that it isn't really an MRI...

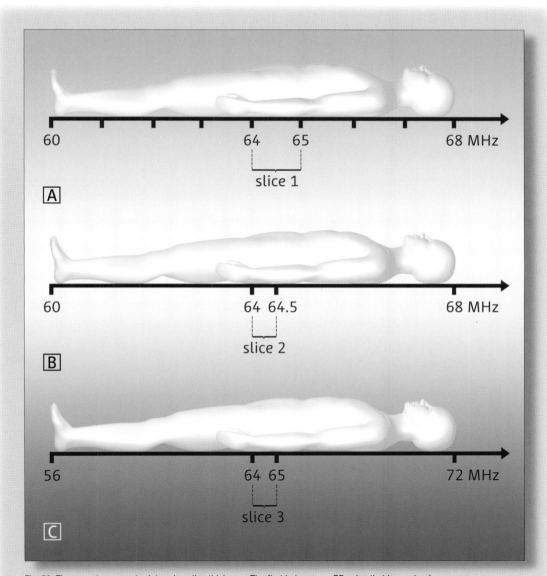

Fig. 58: There are two ways to determine slice thickness. The first is to use an RF pulse that has not only one specific frequency, but a certain range of frequencies, a so-called bandwidth. If, for example, we send in an RF pulse,
which contains frequencies between 64 and 65 MHz, protons in slice 1 will be influenced by the RF pulse.
When the RF pulse only contains frequencies between 64 MHz and 64.5 MHz, thus has a smaller bandwidth, slice 2,
which is half as thick as slice 1, will be imaged.
When there is more difference in magnetic field strength between the level of the feet and the head, i.e. the
magnetic gradient is steeper, the resulting slice will be thinner, even though the RF pulse bandwidth is the same.
This is illustrated in (C), where the magnetic field strength varies more between the feet and the head than in (A);
the corresponding resonant frequencies are 56 to 72 MHz in (C) vs. 60 to 68 MHz in (A). Using the same RF pulse
containing frequencies from 64 to 65 MHz results in imaging of a thinner slice 3 in (C) than in (A).

Where does the signal come from?

Now we have selected position and thickness of our slice. But how can we find out, from what point of our slice a certain signal is coming from – information that we must have to construct an

image? The trick is similar to the slice selecting gradient, which is turned on only during application of the RF pulse.

After the RF pulse is sent in, all protons in the slice precess with the same frequency.

We now apply another gradient field which – in our example – decreases from left to right. So the precession frequency of the protons

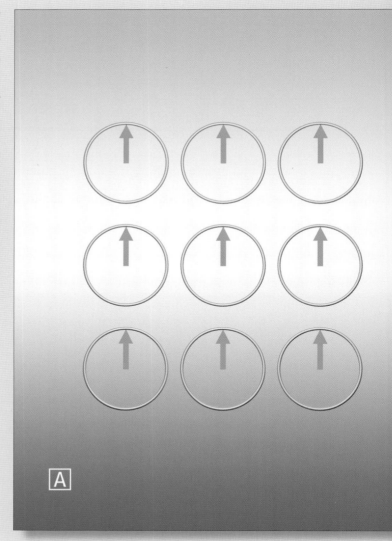

Fig. 59: To determine where in a certain slice a signal comes from, we use a magnetic gradient field. In (A), nine protons in the same slice are depicted. They precess in phase with the same frequency, after the RF pulse is sent in. A magnetic gradient field is then superimposed on the external field, which in (B) decreases in strength from left to right. The protons in the three columns now experience different magnetic fields, and thus give off their signals with different frequencies (e.g. 65, 64 and 63 MHz). The corresponding magnetic gradient is called **the frequency encoding gradient**. We now can tell from which column a signal comes from, but still cannot pinpoint the exact place of origin.

will also decrease from left to right (in our example, the precession frequencies are 65, 64 and 63 MHz, respectively).

The result is that the protons in the different columns emit their signals with these different frequencies. The gradient applied is thus called the **frequency encoding gradient**. However, all protons in one column will still have signals with the same frequency. We now can tell by the frequency from which column a signal comes from, but still cannot pinpoint the exact place of origin in a particular column. As this is not enough spatial information, we have to do something else.

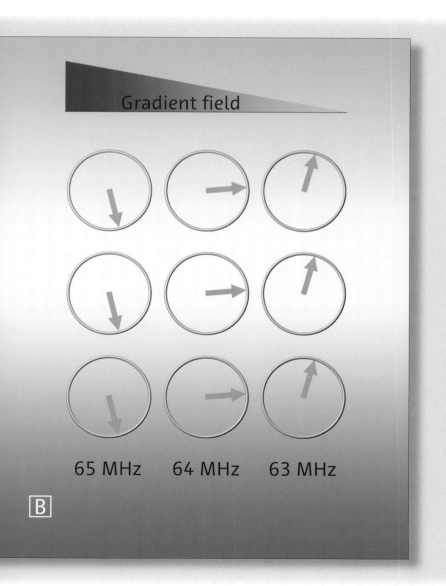

Gradient field

65 MHz   64 MHz   63 MHz

B

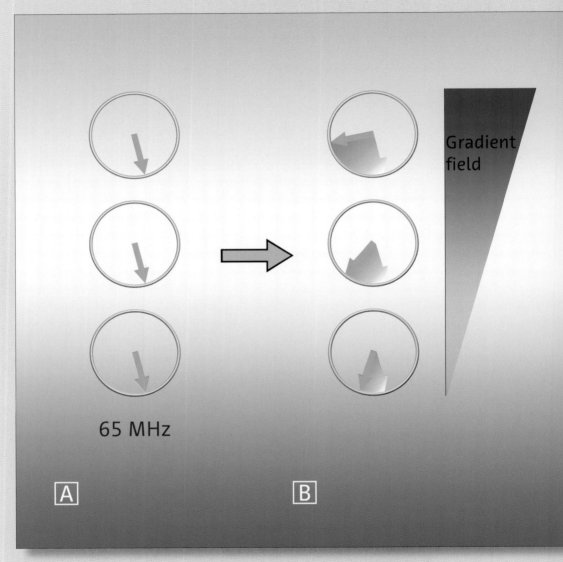

Fig. 60: To find out where in a column with the same frequency a certain signal comes from, we use an additional gradient. In (A), the column with the precession frequency of 65 MHz from figure 59 is depicted. We now switch on a gradient field, which is stronger at the top than at the bottom of the column for a very short time (B). The proton at the top thus precesses faster than the one in the middle, which in turn precesses faster than the proton at the bottom. This difference in precessing frequency only lasts for a very short time; when the gradient is switched off, all protons experience the same magnetic field again, thus have the same 65 MHz precession

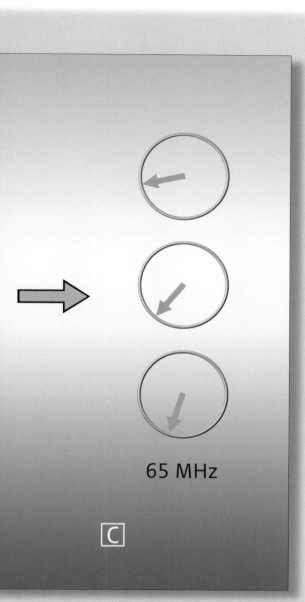

65 MHz

C

frequency again (C). However, now we have a little difference among these protons: even though they precess with the same frequency again, they are a little out of phase, and consequently give off signals of the same frequency, which are different in phase and, because of this, can be differentiated. The corresponding gradient is called the **phase encoding gradient**.

Theoretically, we could use the same trick with the magnetic gradient again. This, however, causes some practical difficulties, e.g. this may result in two points at different locations having the same frequency. To solve the problem, something different is done, which is illustrated in figure 60.

In figure 60, we just look at the protons of one column from figure 59, the 65 MHz column. The protons are in phase after the RF pulse "whipping". Now we apply a magnetic gradient along this column for a short time. This causes the protons to speed up their precession, according to the strength of the magnetic field to which they are being exposed. In our example (figure 60B), the proton at the top thus precesses faster than the one in the middle, which in turn precesses faster than the proton at the bottom.

When this short gradient is switched off, all the protons of the column experience the same magnetic field again, and thus have the same precession frequency. However, there is an important difference: Formerly, the protons (and their signals) were in phase. Now the protons and their signals still have the same frequency, but they are out of phase. (This can be viewed as if their magnetic vectors come by the antenna at different times.)

As the gradient which we used causes protons to precess in different phases, it is called the **phase encoding gradient**.

How this phase encoding actually works is too complicated for a basic introduction.

For here it is enough to know that all of these different signals now can be assigned to a certain location in the slice, so we now can reconstruct our image.

Let us repeat:

● We can select a slice to be examined by using a gradient field, which is superimposed on the external magnetic field. Protons along this gradient field are exposed to different magnetic field strengths, and thus have different precessing frequencies. As they have different precession frequencies, we can send in an RF pulse that contains only those frequencies, which excite the protons in the slice we want to image.

● Slice thickness can be altered in two ways: by changing the bandwidth of the RF pulse, or by modifying the steepness of the gradient field.

● The slice selecting gradient is only turned on during the RF pulse.

● To determine the point in a slice from which a certain signal is coming, we use two other gradients, the frequency encoding gradient and the phase encoding gradient.

● The frequency encoding gradient is sent in after the slice selection gradient. In our example, it is applied in the direction of the x-axis. This results in different precession frequencies along the x-axis, and thus different frequencies of the corresponding signals.

● The phase encoding gradient is turned on for a short time after the RF pulse, along the y-axis in our example. During this short time, the protons along the y-axis precess with different frequencies. When this gradient is switched off, they go back to their former precession frequency, which was the same for all of them. Due to this phase encoding gradient, however, the protons and their signals are now out of phase, which can be detected.

With all this frequency and phase information we can now assign a certain signal to a specific location which results in our MR image (... finally!).

A few more basics

So far we have discussed just about every important aspect of MR basics. But: why have we always talked only about the proton, the hydrogen nucleus? What about other nuclei?

As you recall, atoms have a nucleus made up by **protons** and **neutrons**. An exception is the **hydrogen** nucleus, which only consists of one proton. And when we talk about the proton, we talk about the hydrogen nucleus, as both are the same (the terms proton and hydrogen nucleus can thus be used interchangeably). The hydrogen nucleus is best for MR imaging, as hydrogen occurs in large abundance throughout the body. Hydrogen also gives the best signal among the nuclei: from an equal number of different nuclei in the same magnetic field, hydrogen gives the most intense signal. All of the routine MR imaging is proton/hydrogen imaging nowadays. However, research is being done on the use of other nuclei, like **sodium**.

Can we use all other nuclei for imaging?

The answer is no. There are two important pre-conditions both of which must be fulfilled.

● Firstly, we can only use nuclei that have a spin.

This can be easily explained: as we saw at the beginning, the protons were spinning around, and thus their electrical charge was also spinning, moving. And the moving electrical charge was the current that caused the magnetic field of the proton, which was the basis for everything. If it weren't for the spin, there would be no magnetic field.

● Secondly, the nucleus must have an odd number of protons (and neutrons, but this will go into too much physics, so we will only talk about the protons). Why an odd number? Just think about the proton as a little bar magnet. If you have a nucleus with two (or any other even number) protons, these little bar magnets would cling together like any other magnets (opposite poles attract).

The result: their magnetic moments would cancel each other out. If we have a nucleus with an odd number of protons, e.g. three, pairs of protons will still cling together and neutralize each other. However, there will always be one proton left that still has a magnetic moment. Nuclei with odd numbers of protons thus have a magnetic moment, and can principally be used for MRI.

Examples are: **carbon-13**, **fluorine-19**, **sodium-23**, **phosphorus-31**.

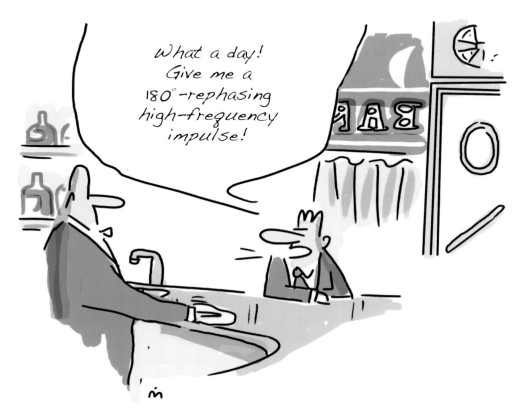

MR Hardware – an overview

Let us have a look at some hardware. The most important part of the MR machine is the main magnet, which has to be pretty strong to allow MR imaging. The strength of a magnet is given in **Tesla** or Gauss, where 1 Tesla = 10,000 **Gauss**.

Gauss was a German mathematician, who was the first to measure the geomagnetic field of the earth. Tesla is considered to be the "father" of the alternating current. He was a peculiar fellow, having refused to share the Nobel prize with the inventor Thomas Edison in the early 1900s.

Magnets used for imaging mostly have **field strengths** up to 1.5 Tesla, meanwhile also 3 Tesla magnets have become popular (they are referred to as "**high field**", with the term "**ultra-high field**" used for even stronger magnets). Basically, the stronger the magnet, the better the MR signal. Unfortunately, technical problems and image artifacts also increase with **magnetic field strength**. Because of that, only magnets up to 3 Tesla are useful for general clinical work at present.

Just to get an idea about the strength of the MR magnets: the earth's magnetic field is between 0.3 and 0.7 G, the magnet of a refrigerator door has about 100 G = 0.01 T).

The magnetic field of MR magnets has to be very homogeneous, as it directly determines the precession frequency. The **homogeneity** is quoted in terms as **ppm**, part per million, in a defined volume. To calculate this, the difference between maximum and minimum field strength is divided by the average field strength and multiplied by one million. How detrimental even rather small inhomogeneities and thus differences in precession frequency can be, has already been illustrated on page 27. Homogeneity of the magnetic field can be improved by making some electrical or mechanical adjustments, a process called **shimming**.

Types of magnets

In MRI, different types of magnets have been used – here a short description.

Permanent magnets:

Everybody is probably familiar with a permanent magnet. It is that type of magnet that fascinates little kids. This kind of magnet is always magnetic and does not use any energy for work, which are its advantages.

Possible disadvantages are thermal instability, its limited field strength, and its weight (a magnet of 0.3 T may weigh about 100 tons!).

This magnet is only used in low field systems today.

Resistive magnets:

In a **resistive magnet**, an electrical current is passed through a loop of wire and generates a magnetic field. Resistive magnets are therefore also called **electromagnets**. They are only magnetic as long as there is an electrical current flowing through them. Thus, they use electrical energy.

As there is a resistance to the flow of the electricity through the wire, these magnets get warm when in operation, and have to be cooled.

Compared with permanent magnets, they achieve a higher field strength. However, resistive magnets are not very practical with high field strengths, because they create lots of heat that must be dissipated. In general, resistive magnets are no longer of central interest.

Superconducting magnets:

Superconducting magnets are the ones most widely used in MR machines. They also make use of electricity, but they have a special current-carrying conductor. This is cooled down to superconducting temperature (about 4 °K or -269 °C). At this temperature, the current conducting material loses its resistance for electricity. So if you send in an electrical current once, it flows in there permanently, creating a constant magnetic field. So-called **cryogens (helium, nitrogen)** are used for cooling of these magnets, and have to be refilled once in a while.

When for some reason the temperature rises above the **superconducting temperature** in these magnets, there will be a loss of superconductivity (so-called **quench**), and sudden resistance to the flow of electricity. This results in rapid heat production, which causes cryogens to boil off rapidly (these leave the system via the so-called **quench lines**). Advantages of superconducting magnets are high magnetic field strength and excellent magnetic field homogeneity. (This is in the order of 10-50 ppm over a region 45 cm in diameter). High field strength and **field homogeneity** facilitate very detailed and fast studies, and allow for spectroscopy.

Disadvantages of the superconducting magnets are their relatively high costs, and use of rather expensive cryogens.

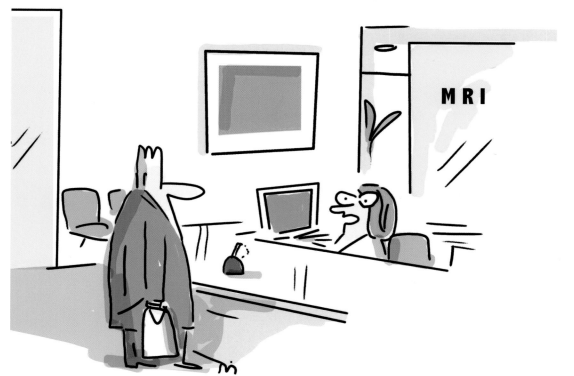

Your insurance card, please. And do you have your protons with you?

Which is the ideal field strength?
This question is as easy to answer as
the question about the ideal horsepow-
er for a car. Here are some of the pros
and cons:
● higher field strength allows for a better spatial resolution and faster examinations, and may be used for spectroscopy;
● low field systems on the other hand
offer better tissue contrast, are cheaper
in price and in operating costs.
   Most MR units today are 1.5 Tesla systems, with 3.0 Tesla systems becoming increasingly popular.

Another piece of
hardware: the coils

In MRI, radio frequency coils are necessary to send in the RF pulse to excite
the protons, and to receive the resulting signal. Coil technology is extreme-
ly important. The same or different
coils can be used for transmission of
the RF pulse and receiving the signal.
A variety of coils are in use – here just
a few comments.

Volume coils

Volume coils are used in all MR units.
These completely surround the part of
the body that is to be imaged. These
volume coils should be close to the size
of the subject.
   The **body coil** is a permanent part of
the scanner, and surrounds the patient.
It is important, as it is the transmitter
for all types of examinations. It also re-
ceives the signal when larger parts of
the body are imaged. Head coils, the
most frequently used dedicated coil
type, may act as receiver coil (with the
body coil transmitting the RF pulses),
or may transmit the RF pulses as well
(so-called transmit-receive coils).

Gradient coils

Gradient coils are used to systemati-
cally vary the magnetic field by pro-
ducing additional linear electromagnetic fields, thus making slice selection and spatial information possible.
As we have three dimensions in space,
there are three sets of gradient coils. As
these coils bang against their anchor-
ing devices, they are the cause of noise
that you can hear during an MR examination.

Surface coils

Surface coils are placed directly on
the area of interest, and have different
shapes corresponding to the part to be
examined.
   They are usually receiver coils only,
most of the received signal coming from
tissues nearby; deeper structures cannot
be examined with these coils. As with
the **head coils**, the RF pulse is transmit-
ted by the body coil in these cases.

Shim coils

As we have already mentioned in con-
nection with the magnets, magnetic
fields have inhomogeneities. Better homogeneity can be achieved by electrical and mechanical adjustments. For
this process, which is called shimming,
the **shim coils** are used.

Why do MR units require
special facilities?

As the systems usually weigh a lot,
there are certain static requirements to
be met. However, there are additional
important factors.
   The strong magnetic field of the MR
system extends beyond the magnet.
Naturally, the magnetic field can attract (even very heavy!) metallic objects and transform them into projec-
tiles! So these have to stay outside the

examination room. Also the magnetic field influences mechanical and electrical devices, like computers, monitors, pacemakers and X-ray units – so such devices must be kept at a certain distance away from the MR unit.

On the other hand, there are also external influences. The whole air is full of radio waves – just think about all the stations which you can receive on your radio. To prevent interference between outside radio waves and those sent from the MR unit, the whole system has to be shielded by a **Faraday cage**.

In addition, it has to be taken into account that larger metallic objects, especially when moving (like elevators, cars), can influence the magnetic field of the scanner, and should also be kept away from the MR unit.

MR spectroscopy

MR spectroscopy has been in use for a long time, long before MR was used for imaging. The procedure is used as an analytical tool, as it can identify various chemical states of certain elements without destruction of the sample. Meanwhile, spectroscopy and imaging may be combined (**spectroscopic imaging**). This enables us to obtain in vivo information about the chemistry and metabolism in specific locations, like in the brain, the liver, or even the heart.

As these measurements can be repeated without harm, follow-up studies of cell physiology are possible. This, for example, can be useful in the evaluation of certain diseases and the effects of therapy.

As spectroscopy requires very homogeneous magnets with higher field strengths, it can only be performed with the use of MR units which have superconducting magnets.

If you listen to the music you say you do, your protons are already accustomed to quite a bit!

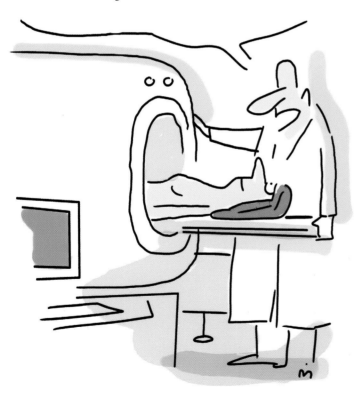

The final review

Now that you have made it up to here, it is our sincere hope that you know a little bit (more?) about MRI. A final review?

Yes, but let us try a different approach this time: take a look at the index on the following pages. Check and see if you understand all of the terms mentioned. If not, refer back to the page numbers listed for a short review.

If you understand all or at least most of it, be happy about it!

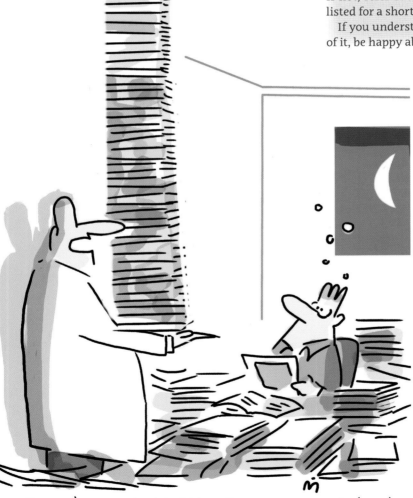

If you've made it this far, a second book shouldn't be any problem at all.

Index

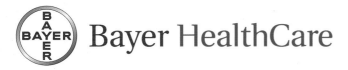

George R.R. Martin
story

John Jos. Miller
sequential adaptation

Ivan Rodriguez
pencils & inks

Ivan Rodriguez
cover

Michael DiPascale, Ivan Rodriguez
chapter breaks, gallery

Digikore Studios
colors

Jaymes Reed
letters

William Christensen **editor-in-chief**
Mark Seifert **creative director**
Jim Kuhoric **managing editor**
David Marks **director of events**
Ariana Osborne **production assistant**

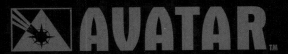

June 2015. Published by Avatar Press, Inc., 515 N. Century Blvd. Rantoul, IL 61866. ©2015 Avatar Press, Inc. In the House of the Worm and all related properties TM & ©2015 George RR Martin. All characters as depicted in this story are over the age of 18. The stories, characters, and institutions mentioned in this magazine are entirely fictional. Printed in Canada.

www.avatarpress.com   www.twitter.com/avatarpress   www.facebook.com/avatarpresscomics

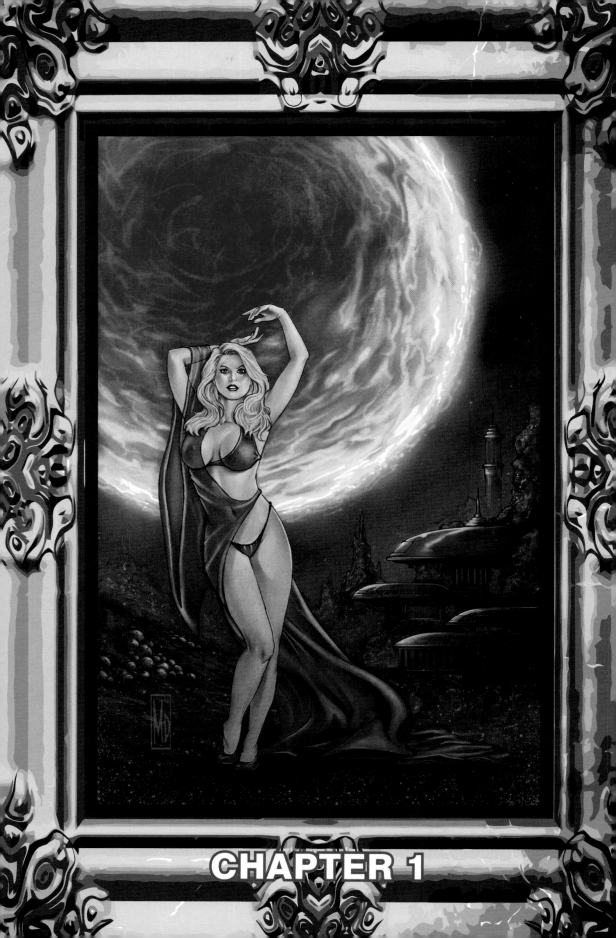

CHAPTER 1

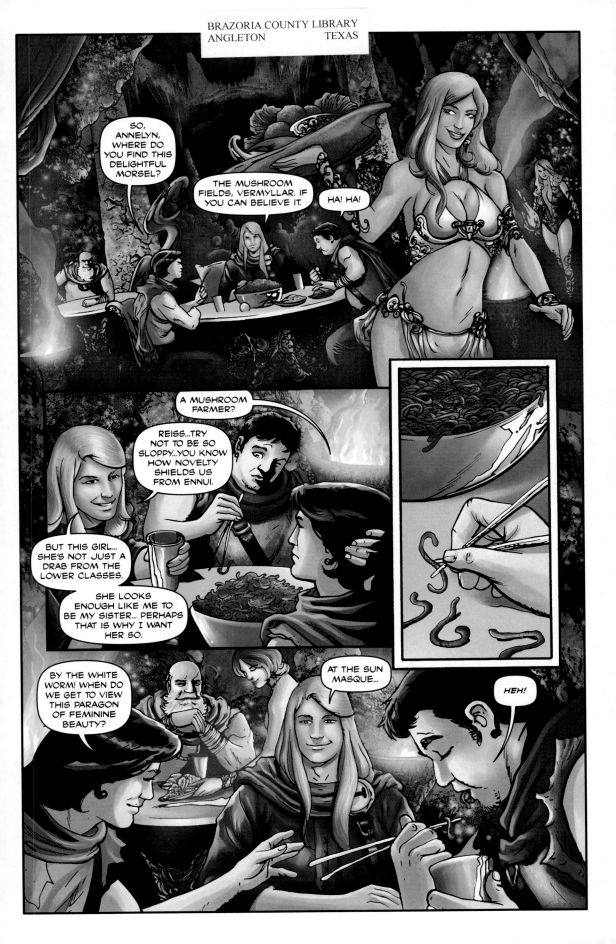

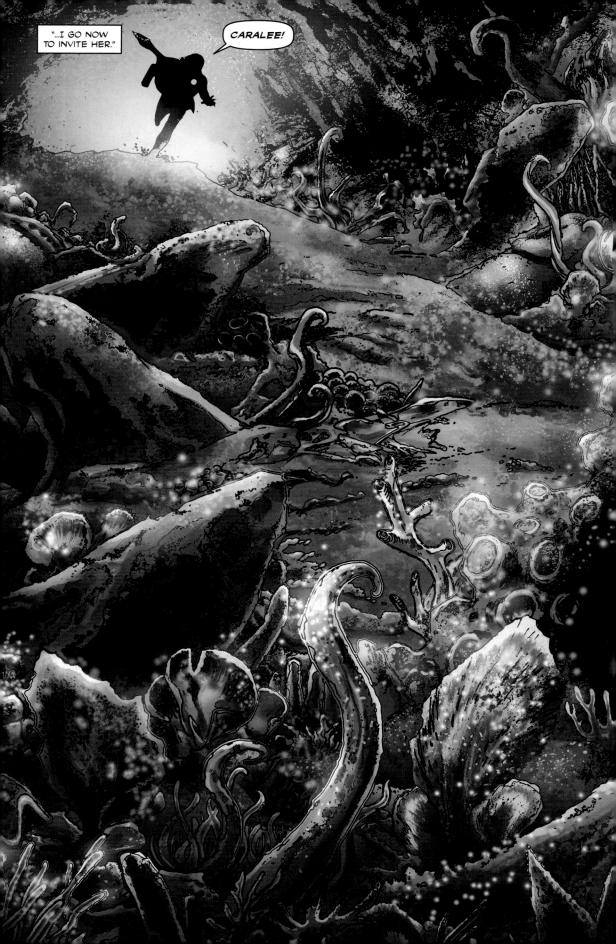

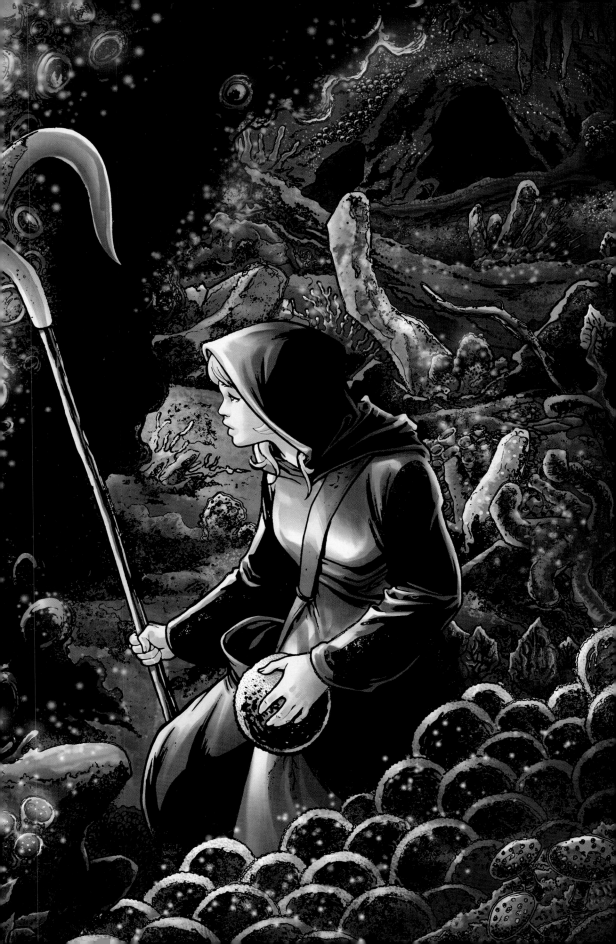

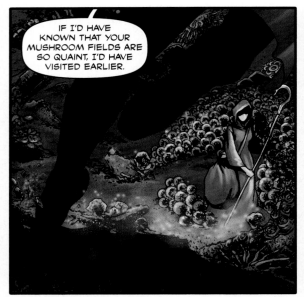

IF I'D HAVE KNOWN THAT YOUR MUSHROOM FIELDS ARE SO QUAINT, I'D HAVE VISITED EARLIER.

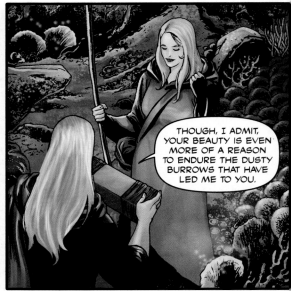

THOUGH, I ADMIT, YOUR BEAUTY IS EVEN MORE OF A REASON TO ENDURE THE DUSTY BURROWS THAT HAVE LED ME TO YOU.

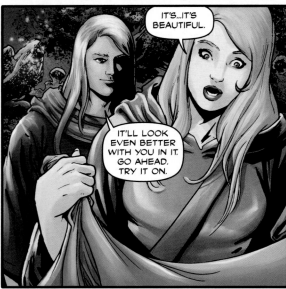

IT'S...IT'S BEAUTIFUL.

IT'LL LOOK EVEN BETTER WITH YOU IN IT. GO AHEAD. TRY IT ON.

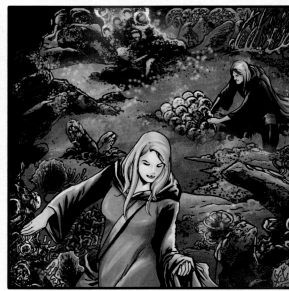

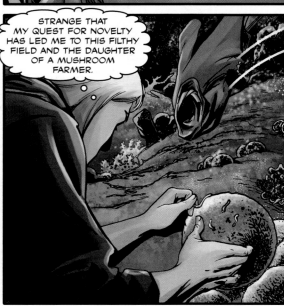

STRANGE THAT MY QUEST FOR NOVELTY HAS LED ME TO THIS FILTHY FIELD AND THE DAUGHTER OF A MUSHROOM FARMER.

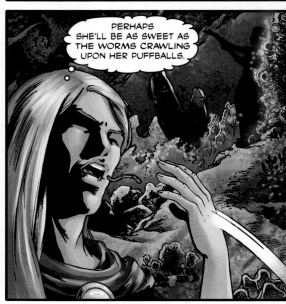

PERHAPS SHE'LL BE AS SWEET AS THE WORMS CRAWLING UPON HER PUFFBALLS.

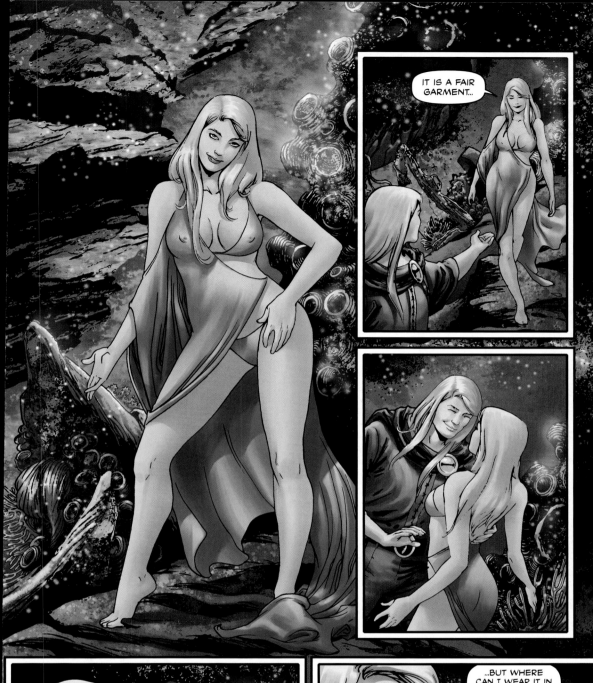

IT IS A FAIR GARMENT...

...BUT WHERE CAN I WEAR IT IN THE MUSHROOM FIELDS?

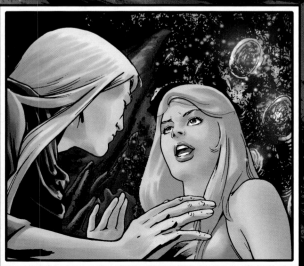

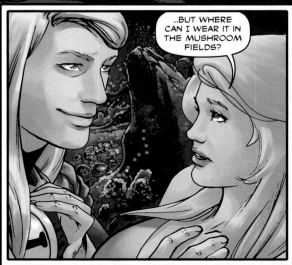

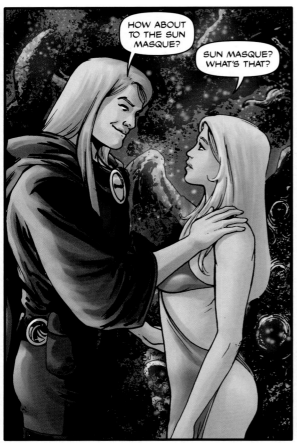

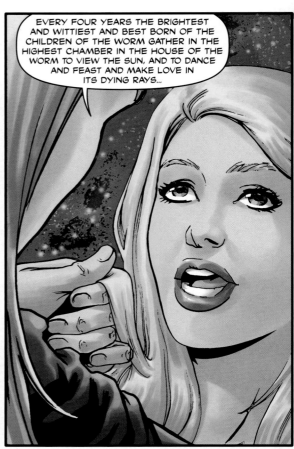

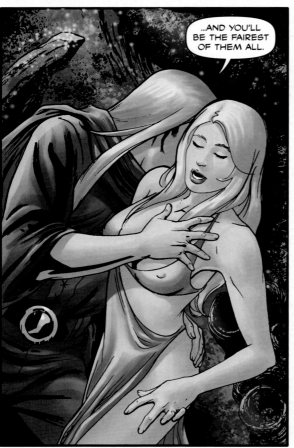

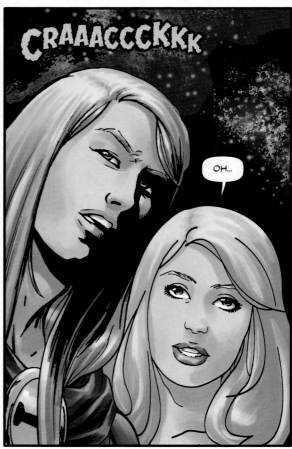

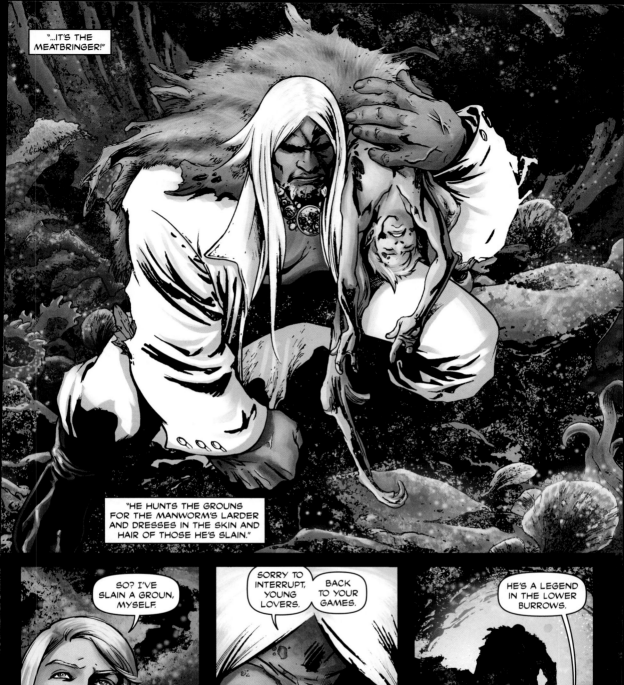

"...IT'S THE MEATBRINGER!"

"HE HUNTS THE GROUNS FOR THE MANWORM'S LARDER AND DRESSES IN THE SKIN AND HAIR OF THOSE HE'S SLAIN."

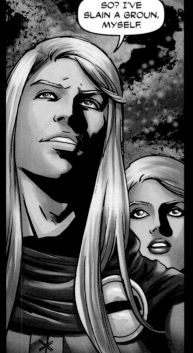

SO? I'VE SLAIN A GROUN, MYSELF.

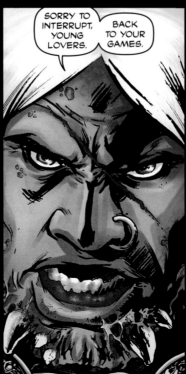

SORRY TO INTERRUPT, YOUNG LOVERS.

BACK TO YOUR GAMES.

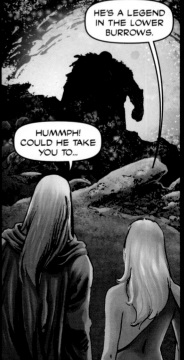

HE'S A LEGEND IN THE LOWER BURROWS.

HUMMPH! COULD HE TAKE YOU TO...

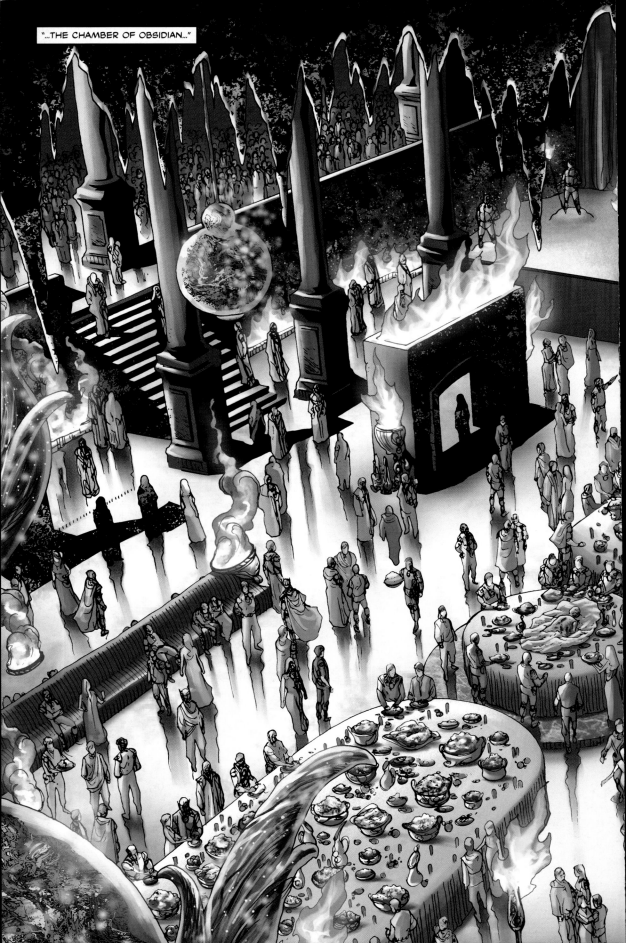

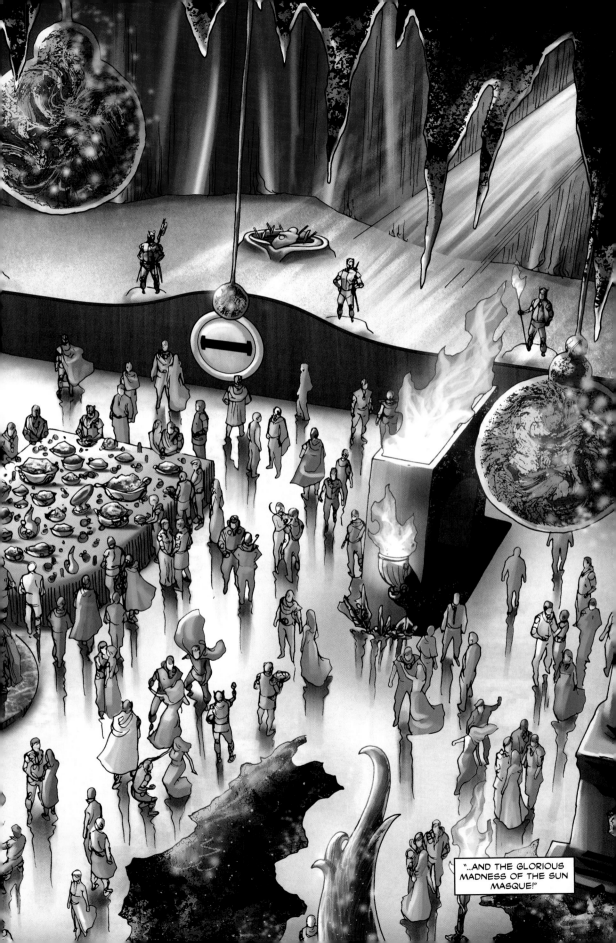

"...AND THE GLORIOUS MADNESS OF THE SUN MASQUE!"

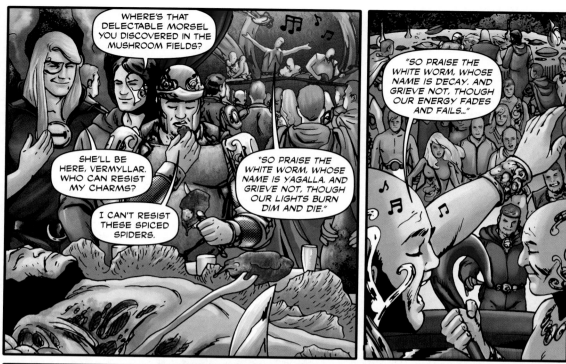

WHERE'S THAT DELECTABLE MORSEL YOU DISCOVERED IN THE MUSHROOM FIELDS?

SHE'LL BE HERE, VERMYLLAR. WHO CAN RESIST MY CHARMS?

I CAN'T RESIST THESE SPICED SPIDERS.

"SO PRAISE THE WHITE WORM, WHOSE NAME IS YAGALLA. AND GRIEVE NOT, THOUGH OUR LIGHTS BURN DIM AND DIE."

"SO PRAISE THE WHITE WORM, WHOSE NAME IS DECAY. AND GRIEVE NOT, THOUGH OUR ENERGY FADES AND FAILS..."

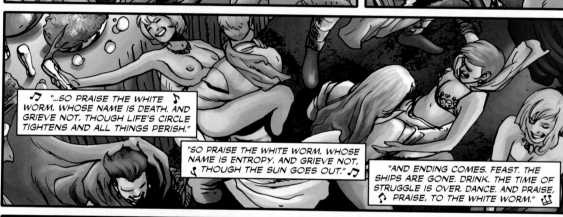

"...SO PRAISE THE WHITE WORM, WHOSE NAME IS DEATH. AND GRIEVE NOT, THOUGH LIFE'S CIRCLE TIGHTENS AND ALL THINGS PERISH."

"SO PRAISE THE WHITE WORM, WHOSE NAME IS ENTROPY. AND GRIEVE NOT, THOUGH THE SUN GOES OUT."

"AND ENDING COMES. FEAST. THE SHIPS ARE GONE. DRINK. THE TIME OF STRUGGLE IS OVER. DANCE. AND PRAISE, PRAISE, TO THE WHITE WORM."

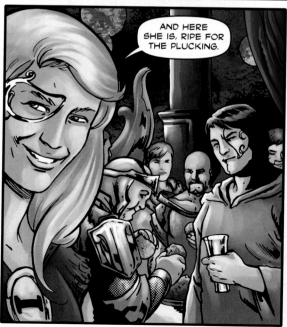

AND HERE SHE IS, RIPE FOR THE PLUCKING.

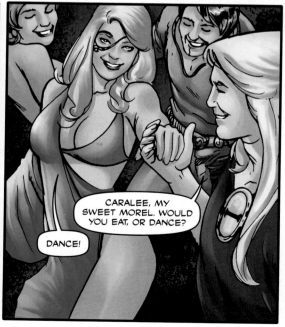

CARALEE, MY SWEET MOREL. WOULD YOU EAT, OR DANCE?

DANCE!

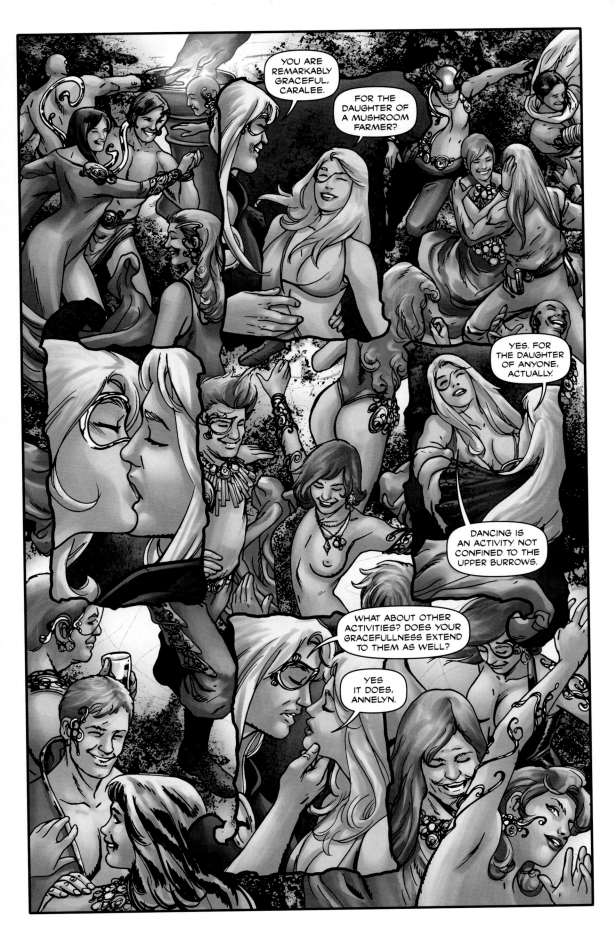

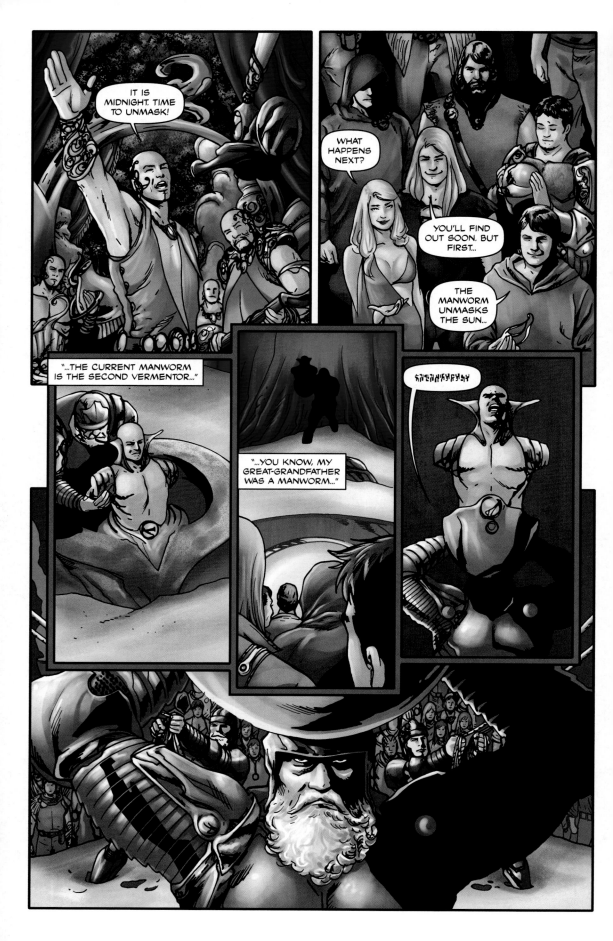

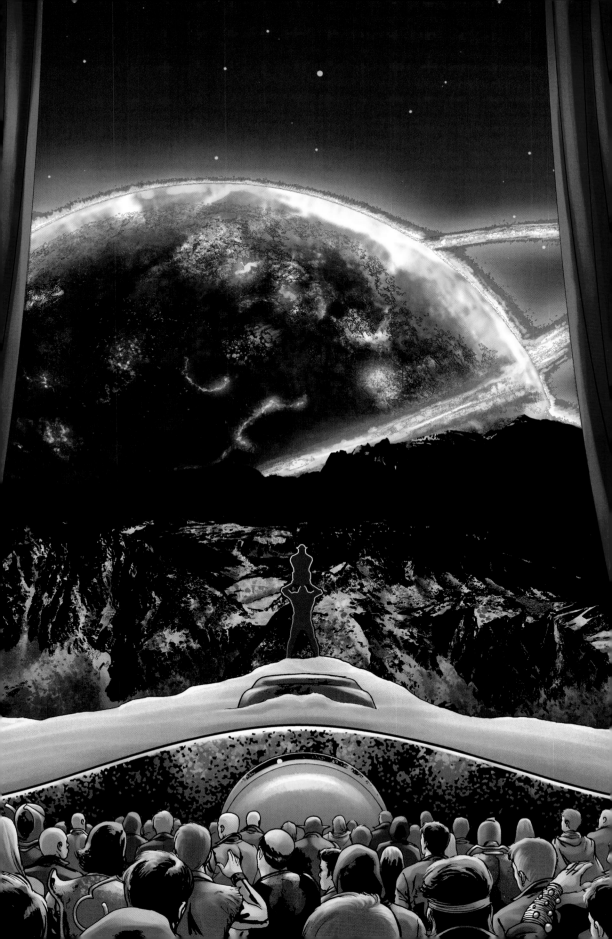

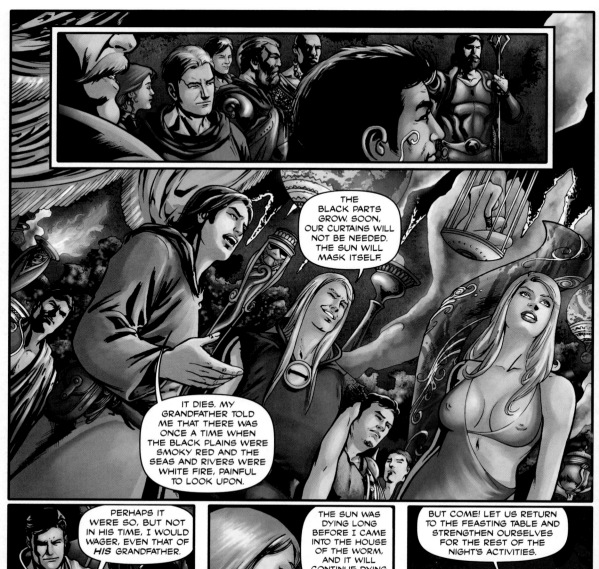

THE BLACK PARTS GROW. SOON, OUR CURTAINS WILL NOT BE NEEDED. THE SUN WILL MASK ITSELF.

IT DIES. MY GRANDFATHER TOLD ME THAT THERE WAS ONCE A TIME WHEN THE BLACK PLAINS WERE SMOKY RED AND THE SEAS AND RIVERS WERE WHITE FIRE, PAINFUL TO LOOK UPON.

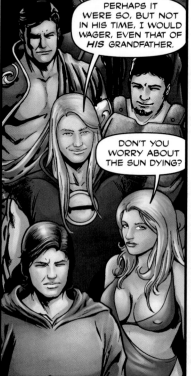

PERHAPS IT WERE SO, BUT NOT IN HIS TIME, I WOULD WAGER, EVEN THAT OF *HIS* GRANDFATHER.

DON'T YOU WORRY ABOUT THE SUN DYING?

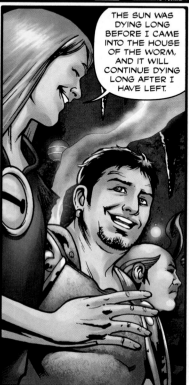

THE SUN WAS DYING LONG BEFORE I CAME INTO THE HOUSE OF THE WORM, AND IT WILL CONTINUE DYING LONG AFTER I HAVE LEFT.

BUT COME! LET US RETURN TO THE FEASTING TABLE AND STRENGTHEN OURSELVES FOR THE REST OF THE NIGHT'S ACTIVITIES.

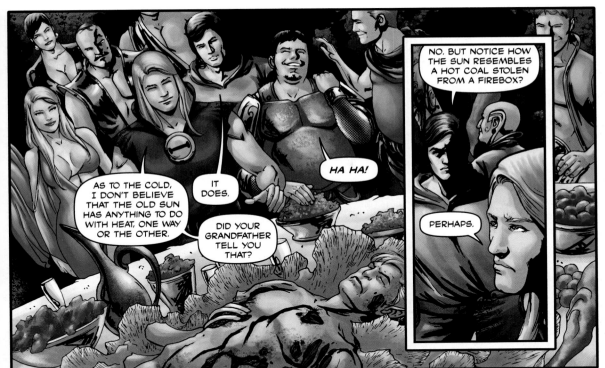

AS TO THE COLD, I DON'T BELIEVE THAT THE OLD SUN HAS ANYTHING TO DO WITH HEAT, ONE WAY OR THE OTHER.

IT DOES.

DID YOUR GRANDFATHER TELL YOU THAT?

HA HA!

NO. BUT NOTICE HOW THE SUN RESEMBLES A HOT COAL STOLEN FROM A FIREBOX?

PERHAPS.

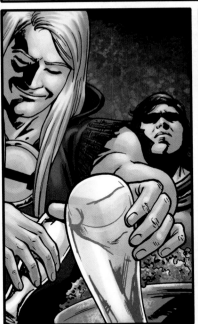

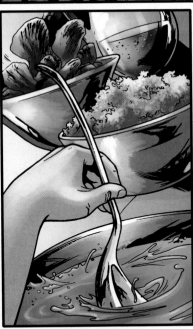

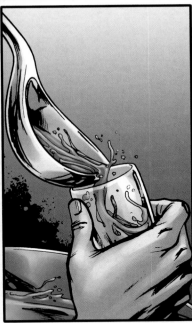

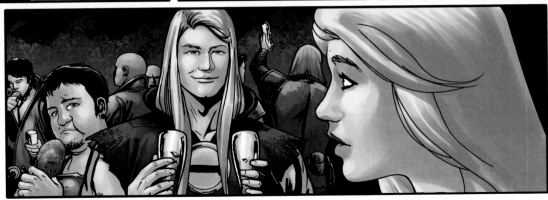

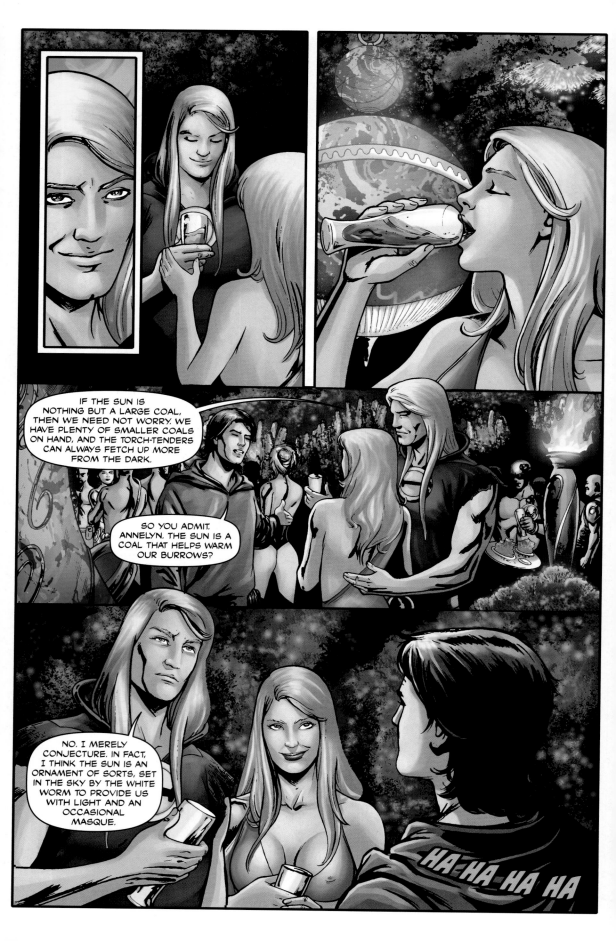

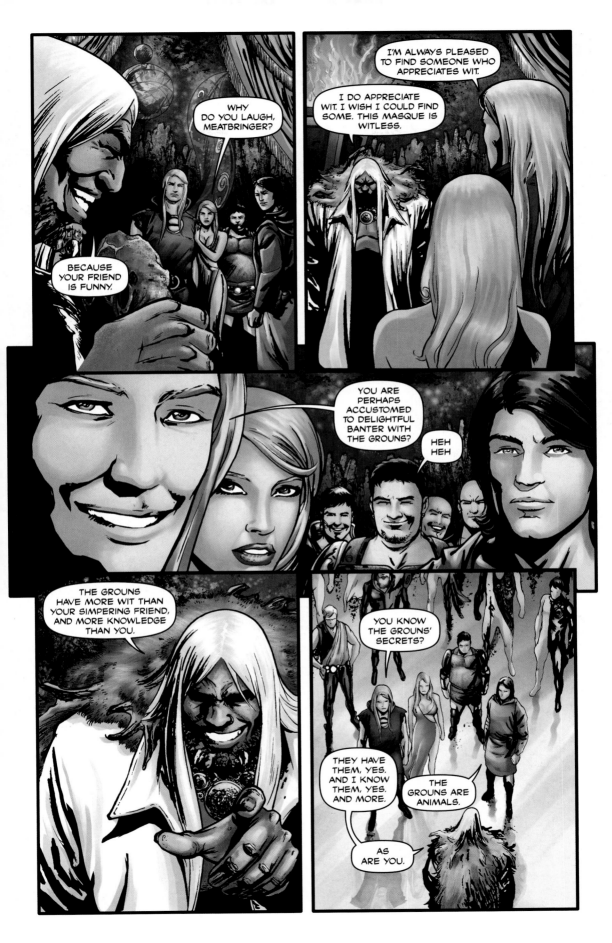

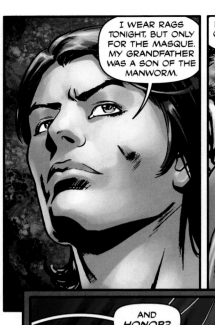

I WEAR RAGS TONIGHT, BUT ONLY FOR THE MASQUE. MY GRANDFATHER WAS A SON OF THE MANWORM.

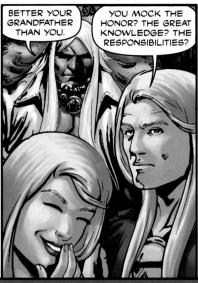

BETTER YOUR GRANDFATHER THAN YOU.

YOU MOCK THE HONOR? THE GREAT KNOWLEDGE? THE RESPONSIBILITIES?

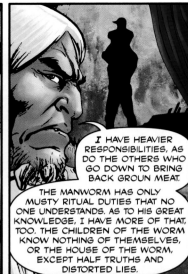

I HAVE HEAVIER RESPONSIBILITIES, AS DO THE OTHERS WHO GO DOWN TO BRING BACK GROUN MEAT.

THE MANWORM HAS ONLY MUSTY RITUAL DUTIES THAT NO ONE UNDERSTANDS. AS TO HIS GREAT KNOWLEDGE, I HAVE MORE OF THAT, TOO. THE CHILDREN OF THE WORM KNOW NOTHING OF THEMSELVES, OR THE HOUSE OF THE WORM, EXCEPT HALF TRUTHS AND DISTORTED LIES.

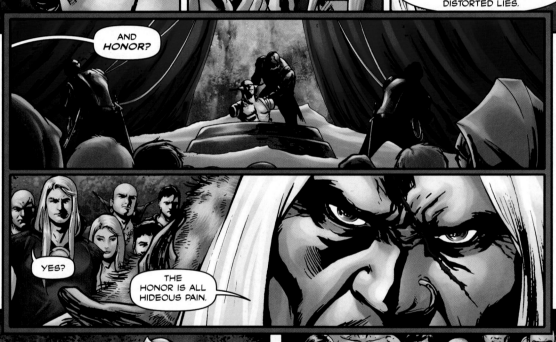

AND *HONOR?*

YES?

THE HONOR IS ALL HIDEOUS PAIN.

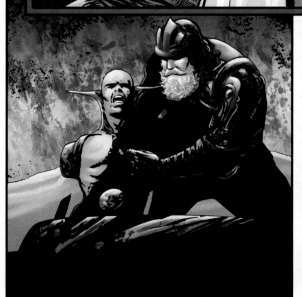

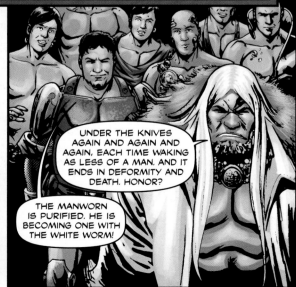

UNDER THE KNIVES AGAIN AND AGAIN AND AGAIN, EACH TIME WAKING AS LESS OF A MAN. AND IT ENDS IN DEFORMITY AND DEATH. HONOR?

THE MANWORN IS PURIFIED. HE IS BECOMING ONE WITH THE WHITE WORM!

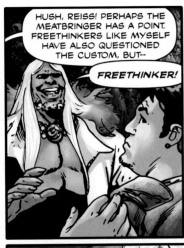

HUSH, REISS! PERHAPS THE MEATBRINGER HAS A POINT. FREETHINKERS LIKE MYSELF HAVE ALSO QUESTIONED THE CUSTOM, BUT--

FREETHINKER!

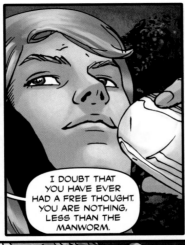

I DOUBT THAT YOU HAVE EVER HAD A FREE THOUGHT. YOU ARE NOTHING, LESS THAN THE MANWORM.

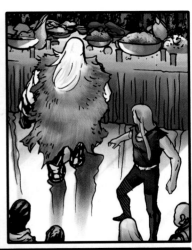

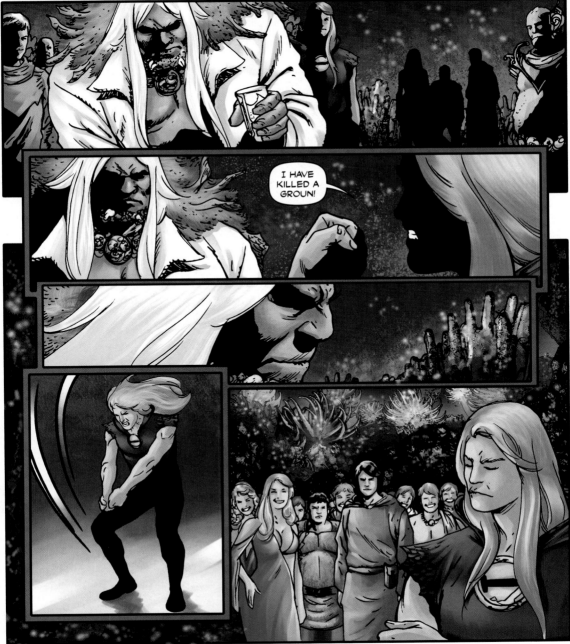

I HAVE KILLED A GROUN!

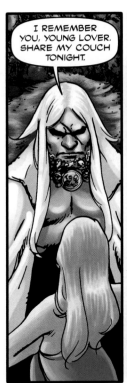

I REMEMBER YOU, YOUNG LOVER. SHARE MY COUCH TONIGHT.

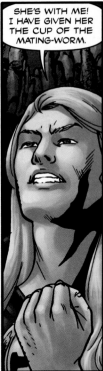

SHE'S WITH ME! I HAVE GIVEN HER THE CUP OF THE MATING-WORM.

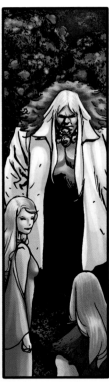

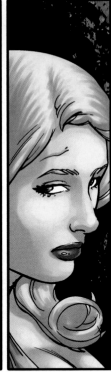

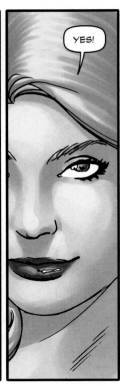

YES!

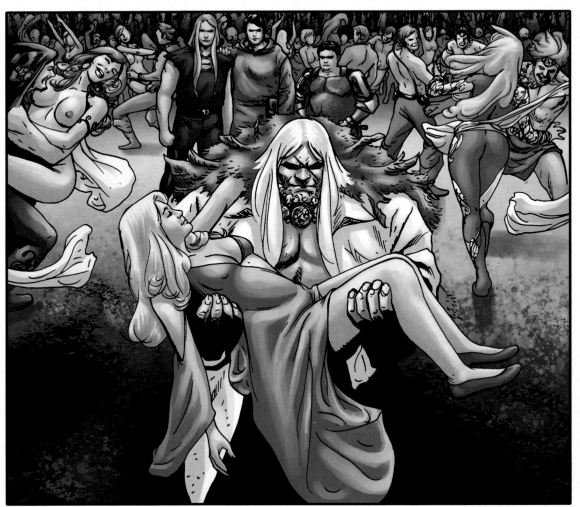

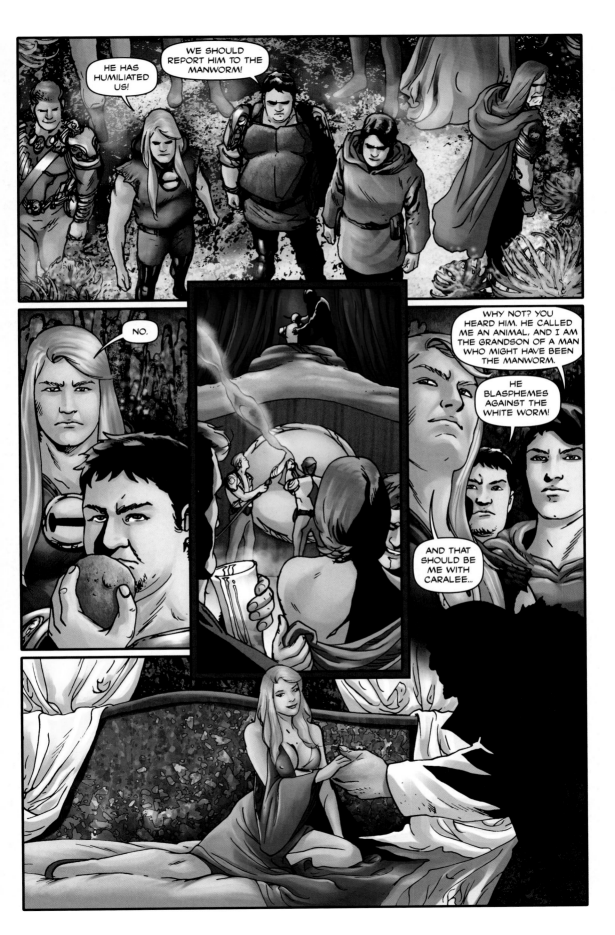

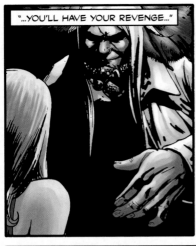

"...YOU'LL HAVE YOUR REVENGE..."

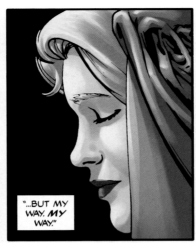

"...BUT MY WAY. *MY WAY.*"

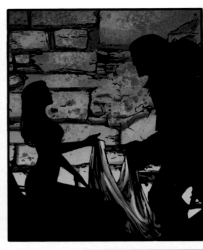

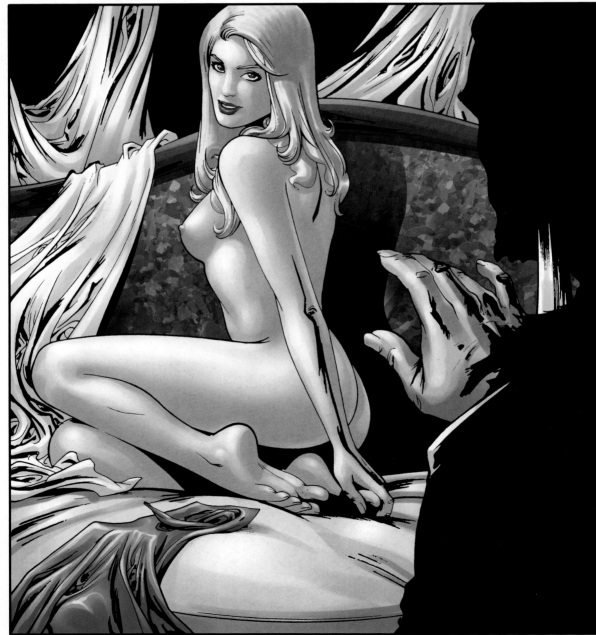

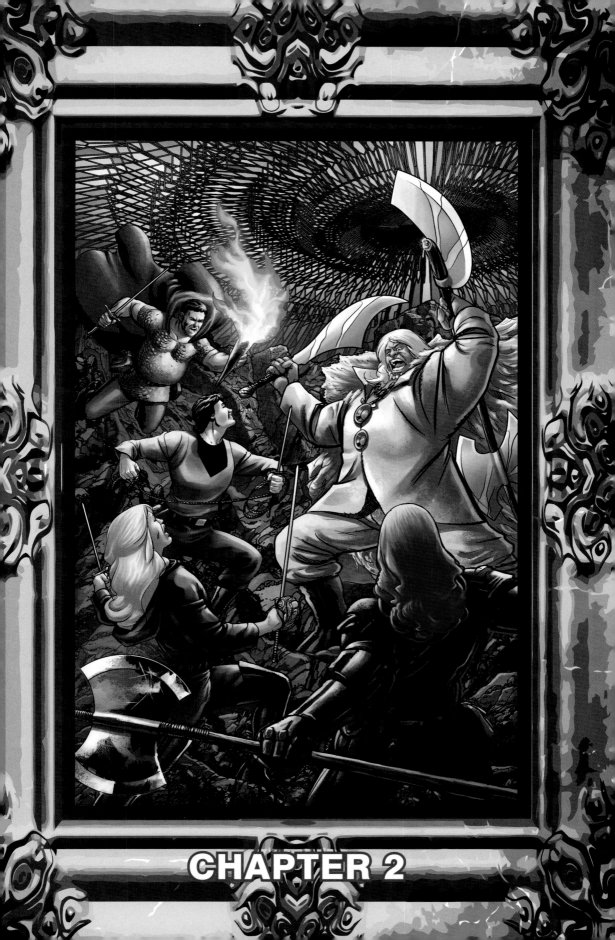

CHAPTER 2

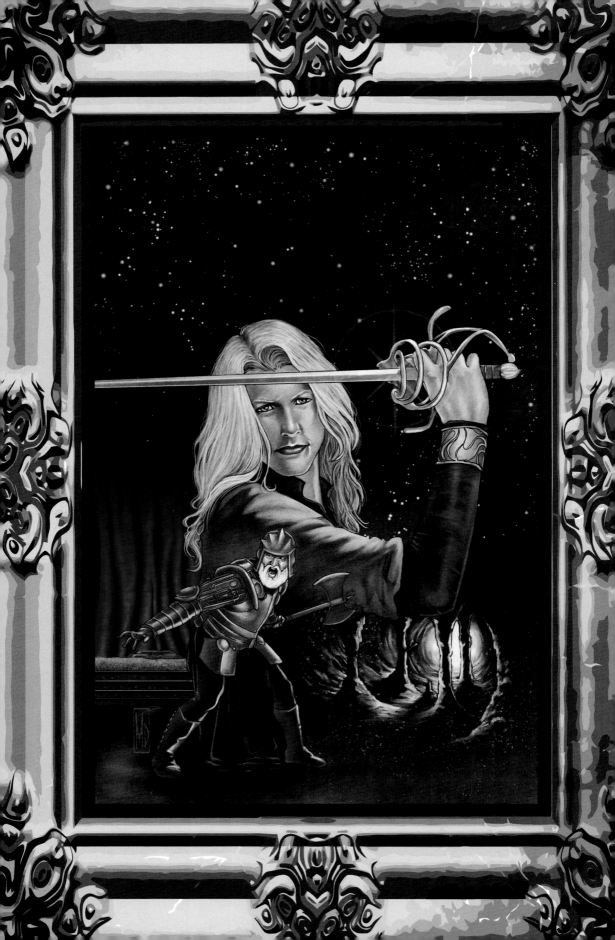

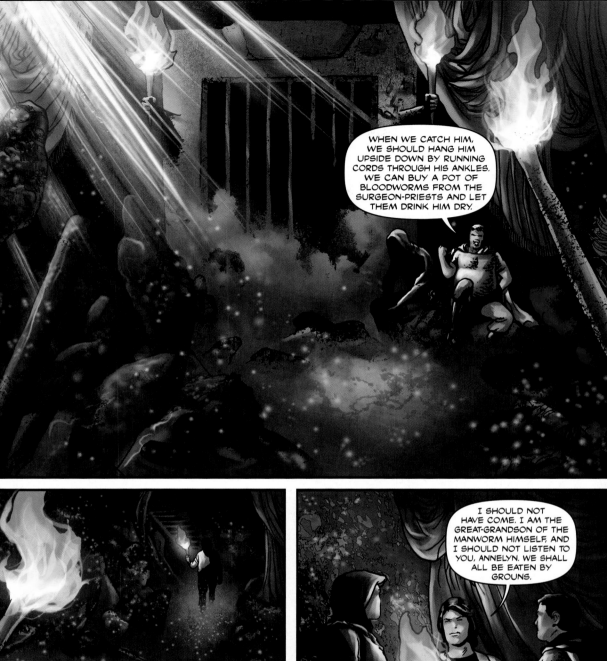

WHEN WE CATCH HIM, WE SHOULD HANG HIM UPSIDE DOWN BY RUNNING CORDS THROUGH HIS ANKLES. WE CAN BUY A POT OF BLOODWORMS FROM THE SURGEON-PRIESTS AND LET THEM DRINK HIM DRY.

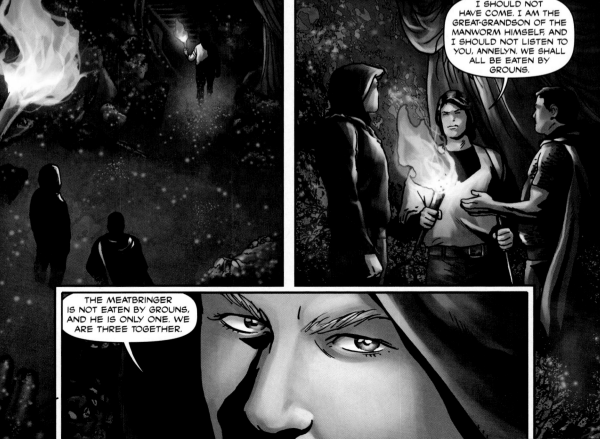

I SHOULD NOT HAVE COME. I AM THE GREAT-GRANDSON OF THE MANWORM HIMSELF, AND I SHOULD NOT LISTEN TO YOU, ANNELYN. WE SHALL ALL BE EATEN BY GROUNS.

THE MEATBRINGER IS NOT EATEN BY GROUNS, AND HE IS ONLY ONE. WE ARE THREE TOGETHER.

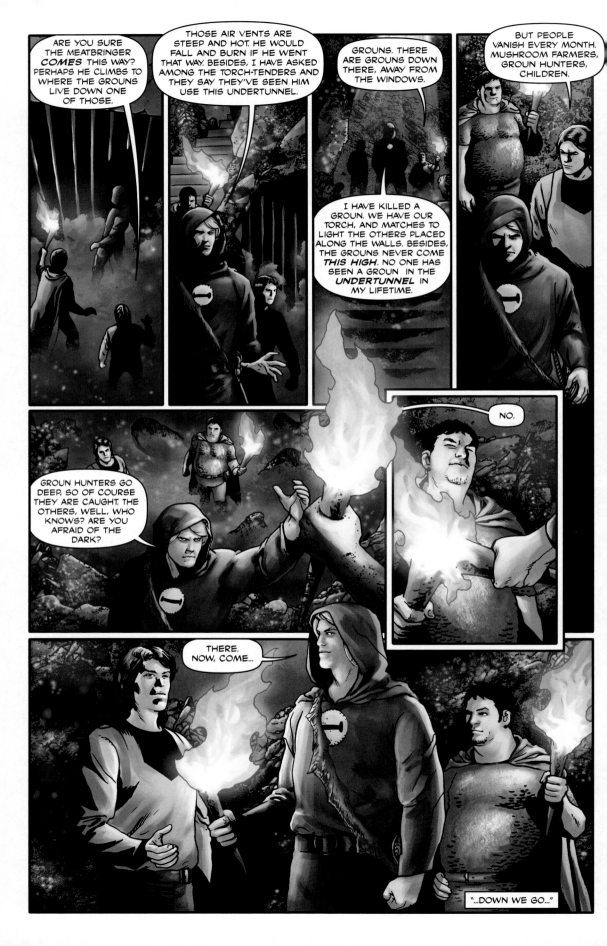

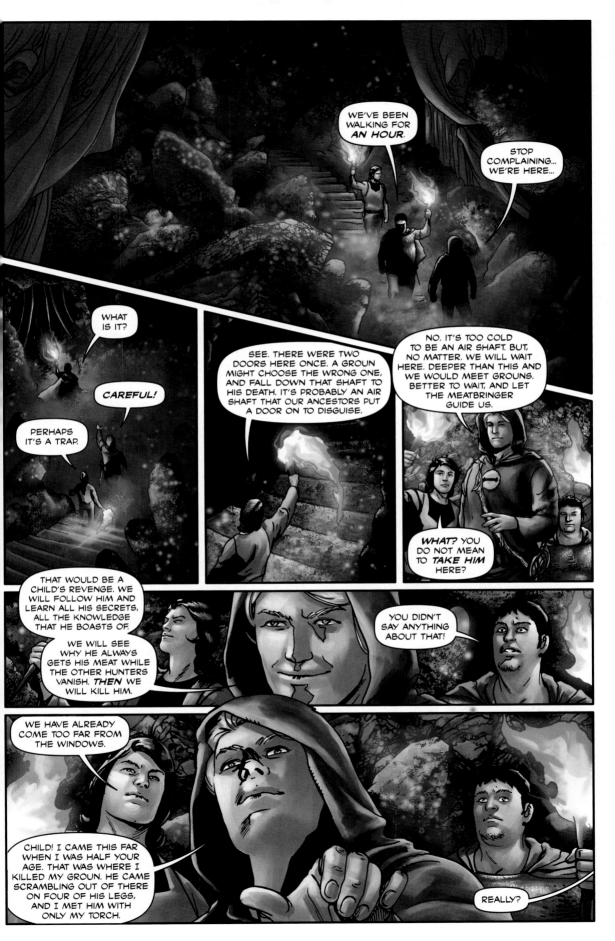

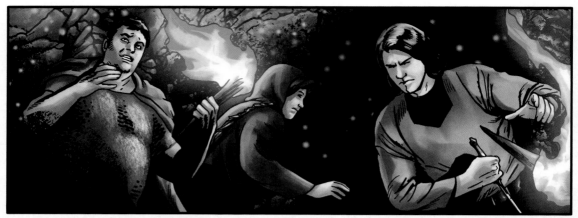

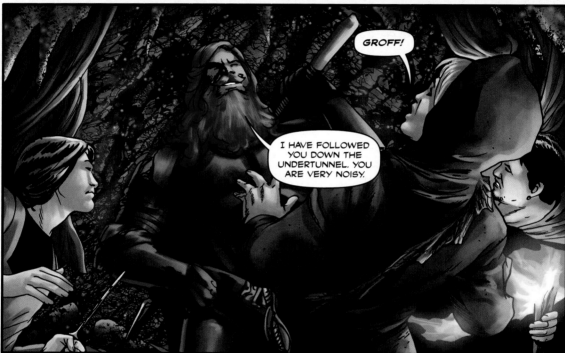

GROFF!

I HAVE FOLLOWED YOU DOWN THE UNDERTUNNEL. YOU ARE VERY NOISY.

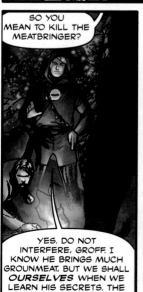

SO YOU MEAN TO KILL THE MEATBRINGER?

YES. DO NOT INTERFERE, GROFF. I KNOW HE BRINGS MUCH GROUNMEAT, BUT WE SHALL *OURSELVES* WHEN WE LEARN HIS SECRETS. THE MANWORM HAS NO CAUSE TO TAKE HIS SIDE.

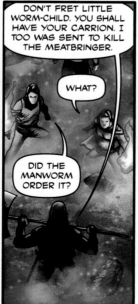

DON'T FRET LITTLE WORM-CHILD. YOU SHALL HAVE YOUR CARRION. I TOO WAS SENT TO KILL THE MEATBRINGER.

WHAT?

DID THE MANWORM ORDER IT?

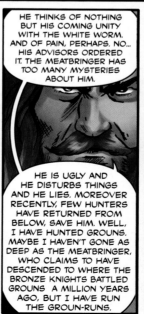

HE THINKS OF NOTHING BUT HIS COMING UNITY WITH THE WHITE WORM, AND OF PAIN, PERHAPS. NO... HIS ADVISORS ORDERED IT. THE MEATBRINGER HAS TOO MANY MYSTERIES ABOUT HIM.

HE IS UGLY AND HE DISTURBS THINGS AND HE LIES. MOREOVER RECENTLY, FEW HUNTERS HAVE RETURNED FROM BELOW, SAVE HIM. WELL, I HAVE HUNTED GROUNS. MAYBE I HAVEN'T GONE AS DEEP AS THE MEATBRINGER, WHO CLAIMS TO HAVE DESCENDED TO WHERE THE BRONZE KNIGHTS BATTLED GROUNS A MILLION YEARS AGO, BUT I HAVE RUN THE GROUN-RUNS.

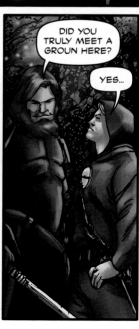

DID YOU TRULY MEET A GROUN HERE?

YES...

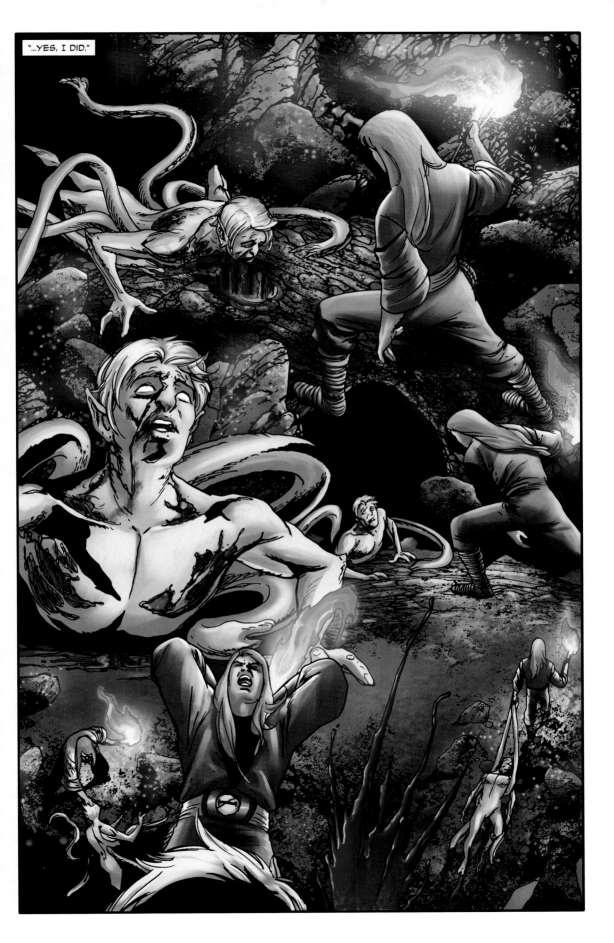

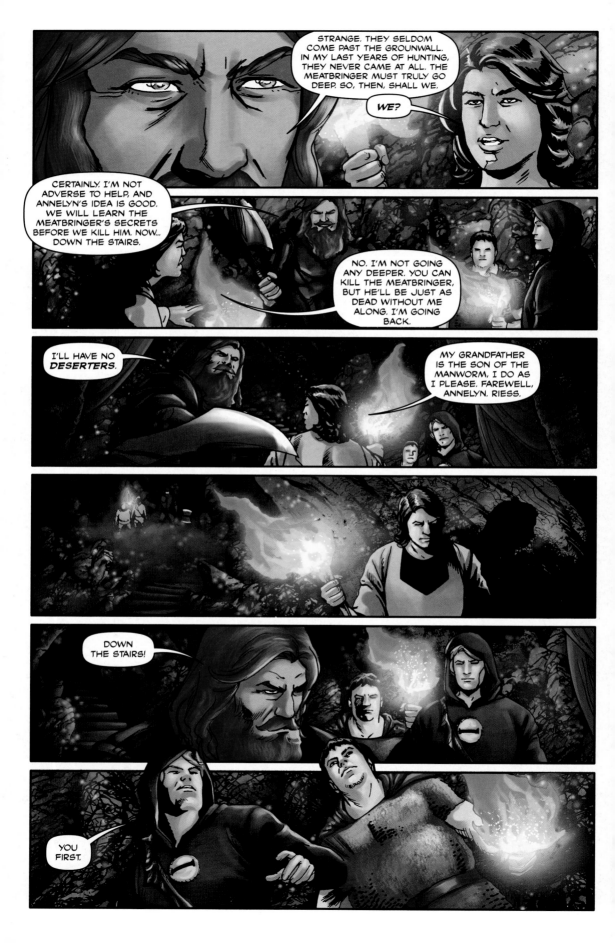

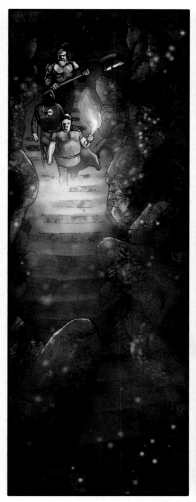
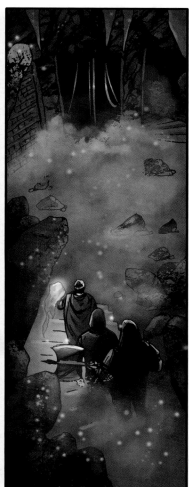
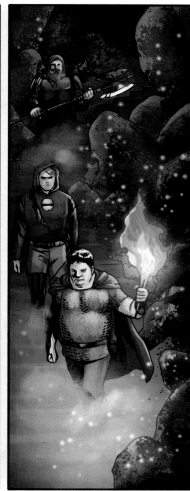
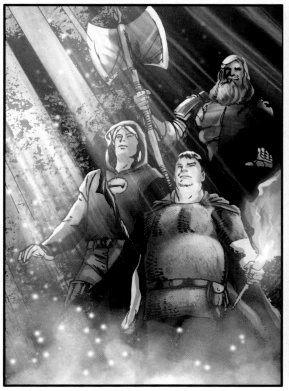
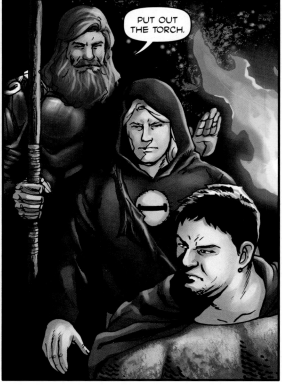

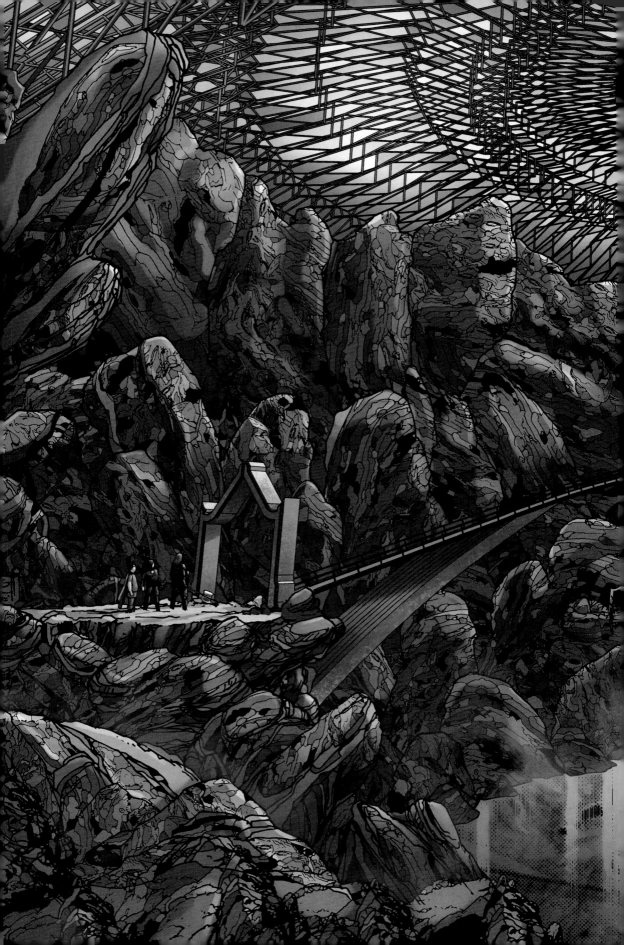

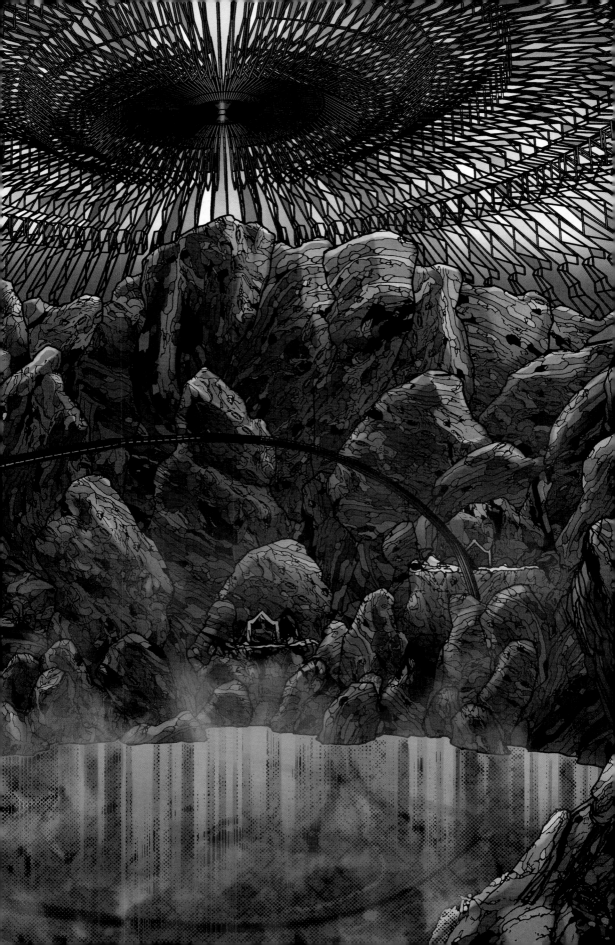

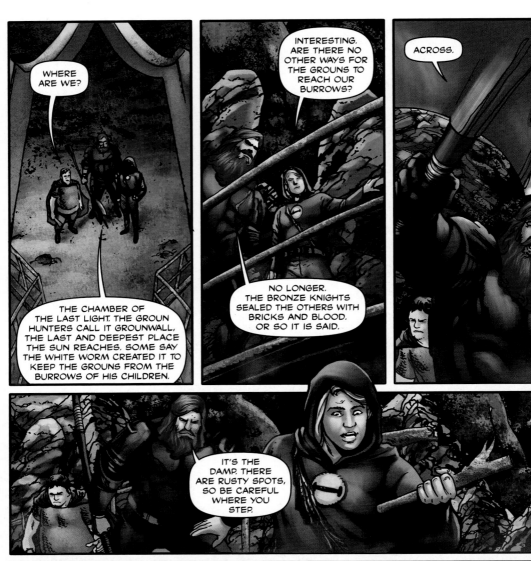
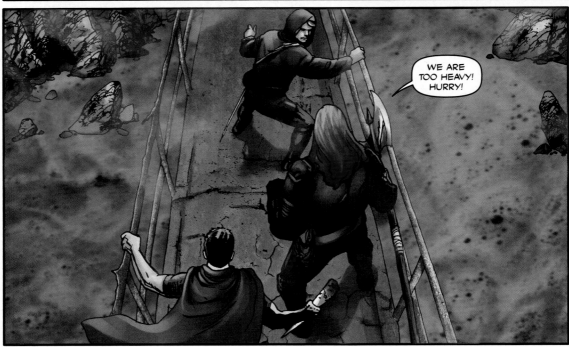

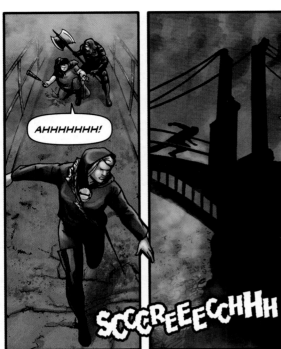

AHHHHHHH!

SCCGREEEECHHH

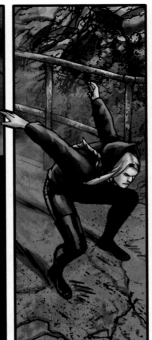

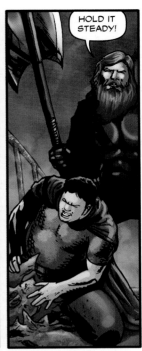

HOLD IT STEADY!

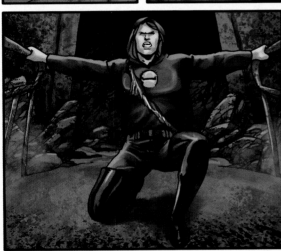

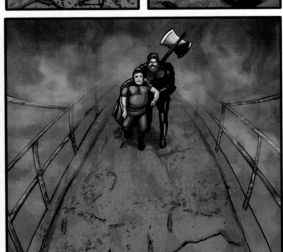

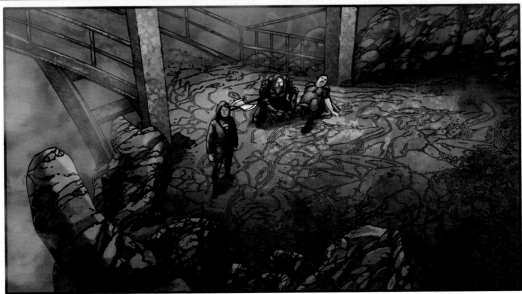

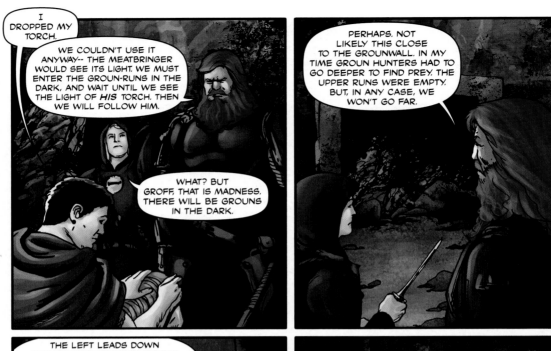

I DROPPED MY TORCH.

WE COULDN'T USE IT ANYWAY-- THE MEATBRINGER WOULD SEE ITS LIGHT. WE MUST ENTER THE GROUN-RUNS IN THE DARK, AND WAIT UNTIL WE SEE THE LIGHT OF *HIS* TORCH. THEN WE WILL FOLLOW HIM.

WHAT? BUT GROFF, THAT IS MADNESS. THERE WILL BE GROUNS IN THE DARK.

PERHAPS. NOT LIKELY THIS CLOSE TO THE GROUNWALL. IN MY TIME GROUN HUNTERS HAD TO GO DEEPER TO FIND PREY. THE UPPER RUNS WERE EMPTY. BUT, IN ANY CASE, WE WON'T GO FAR.

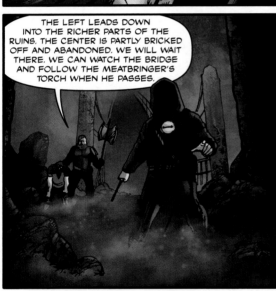

THE LEFT LEADS DOWN INTO THE RICHER PARTS OF THE RUINS. THE CENTER IS PARTLY BRICKED OFF AND ABANDONED. WE WILL WAIT THERE. WE CAN WATCH THE BRIDGE AND FOLLOW THE MEATBRINGER'S TORCH WHEN HE PASSES.

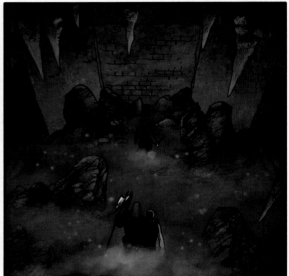

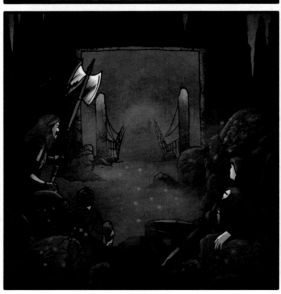

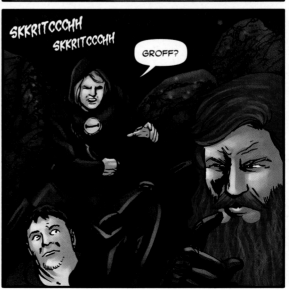

SKKRITCCCHH
SKKRITCCCHH

GROFF?

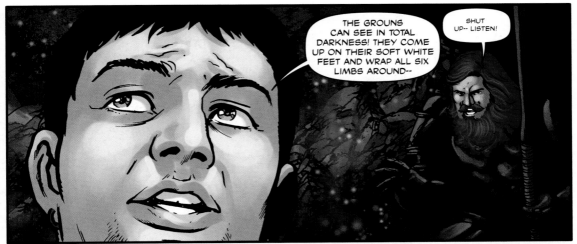

THE GROUNS CAN SEE IN TOTAL DARKNESS! THEY COME UP ON THEIR SOFT WHITE FEET AND WRAP ALL SIX LIMBS AROUND--

SHUT UP-- LISTEN!

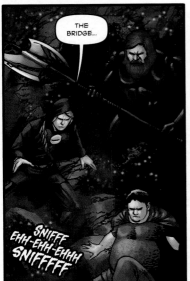

THE BRIDGE...

SNIFFF EHH-EHH-EHHH SNIFFFFF

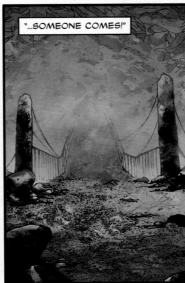

"...SOMEONE COMES!"

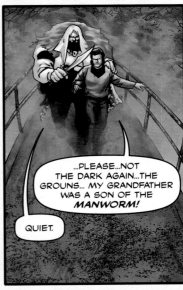

...PLEASE...NOT THE DARK AGAIN...THE GROUNS... MY GRANDFATHER WAS A SON OF THE MANWORM!

QUIET.

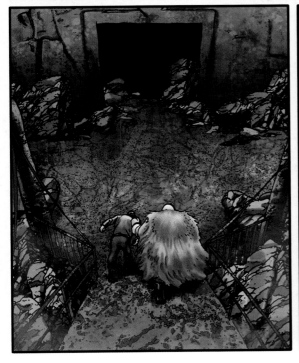

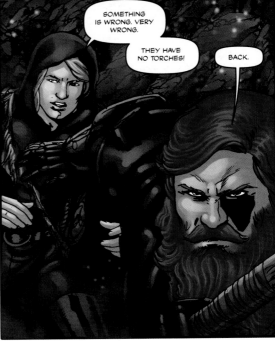

SOMETHING IS WRONG. VERY WRONG.

THEY HAVE NO TORCHES!

BACK.

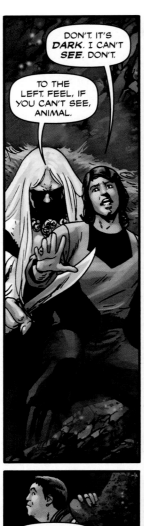

DON'T. IT'S *DARK*. I CAN'T *SEE*. DON'T.

TO THE LEFT. FEEL, IF YOU CAN'T SEE, ANIMAL.

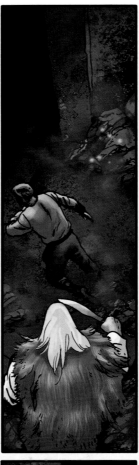

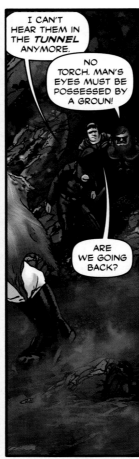

I CAN'T HEAR THEM IN THE *TUNNEL* ANYMORE.

NO TORCH. MAN'S EYES MUST BE POSSESSED BY A GROUN!

ARE WE GOING BACK?

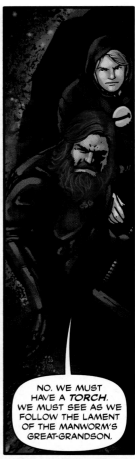

NO. WE MUST HAVE A *TORCH*. WE MUST SEE AS WE FOLLOW THE LAMENT OF THE MANWORM'S GREAT-GRANDSON.

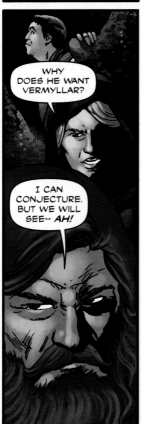

WHY DOES HE WANT VERMYLLAR?

I CAN CONJECTURE. BUT WE WILL SEE-- *AH!*

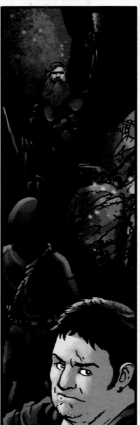

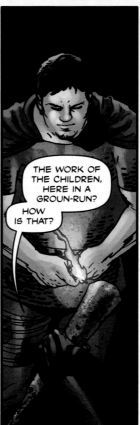

THE WORK OF THE CHILDREN, HERE IN A GROUN-RUN?

HOW IS THAT?

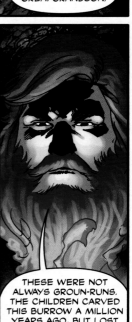

THESE WERE NOT ALWAYS GROUN-RUNS. THE CHILDREN CARVED THIS BURROW A MILLION YEARS AGO, BUT LOST IT IN ANCIENT WARFARE. THE BURROWS THAT HAVE ALWAYS BEEN THE GROUNS' ARE DIFFERENT.

BUT COME-- WE MUST NOT LOSE THEM...

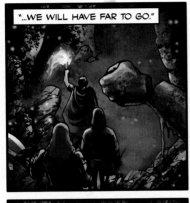

"...WE WILL HAVE FAR TO GO."

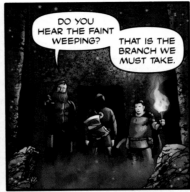

DO YOU HEAR THE FAINT WEEPING?

THAT IS THE BRANCH WE MUST TAKE.

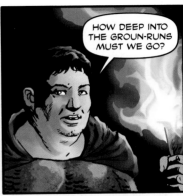

HOW DEEP INTO THE GROUN-RUNS MUST WE GO?

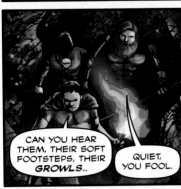

CAN YOU HEAR THEM, THEIR SOFT FOOTSTEPS, THEIR *GROWLS*...

QUIET, YOU FOOL.

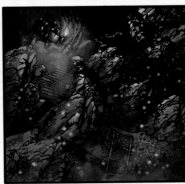

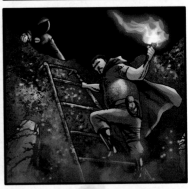

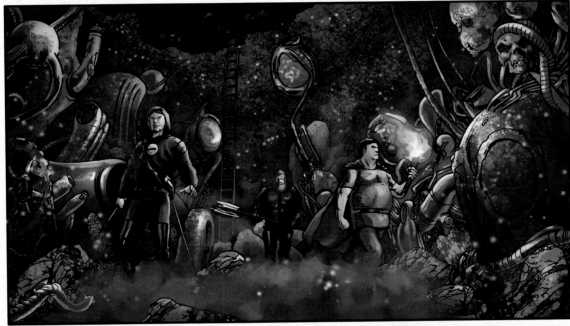

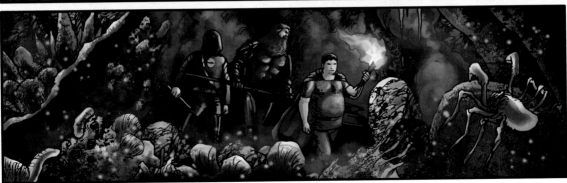

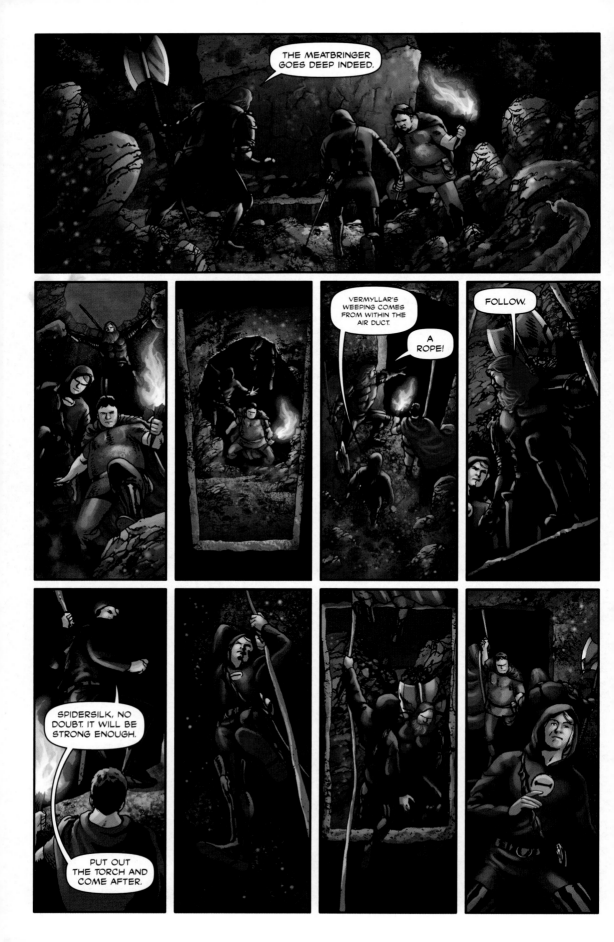

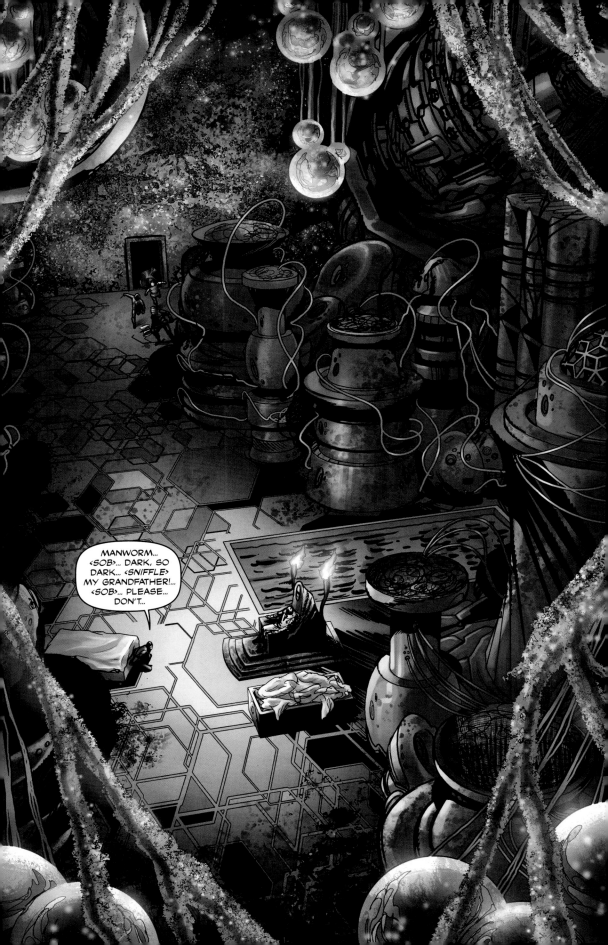

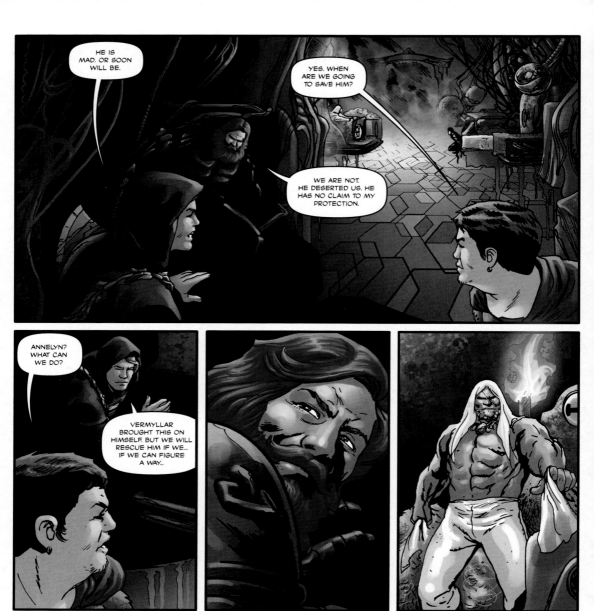

HE IS MAD. OR SOON WILL BE.

YES. WHEN ARE WE GOING TO SAVE HIM?

WE ARE NOT. HE DESERTED US. HE HAS NO CLAIM TO MY PROTECTION.

ANNELYN? WHAT CAN WE DO?

VERMYLLAR BROUGHT THIS ON HIMSELF. BUT WE WILL RESCUE HIM IF WE... IF WE CAN FIGURE A WAY...

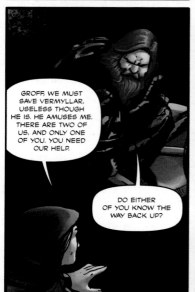

GROFF, WE MUST SAVE VERMYLLAR, USELESS THOUGH HE IS. HE AMUSES ME. THERE ARE TWO OF US, AND ONLY ONE OF YOU. YOU NEED OUR HELP.

DO EITHER OF YOU KNOW THE WAY BACK UP?

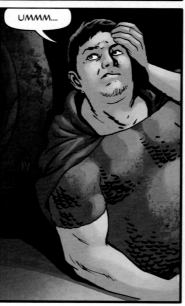

UMMM....

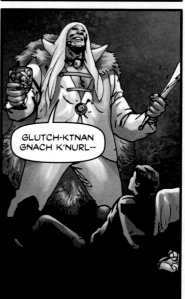

GLUTCH-KTNAN GNACH K'NURL--

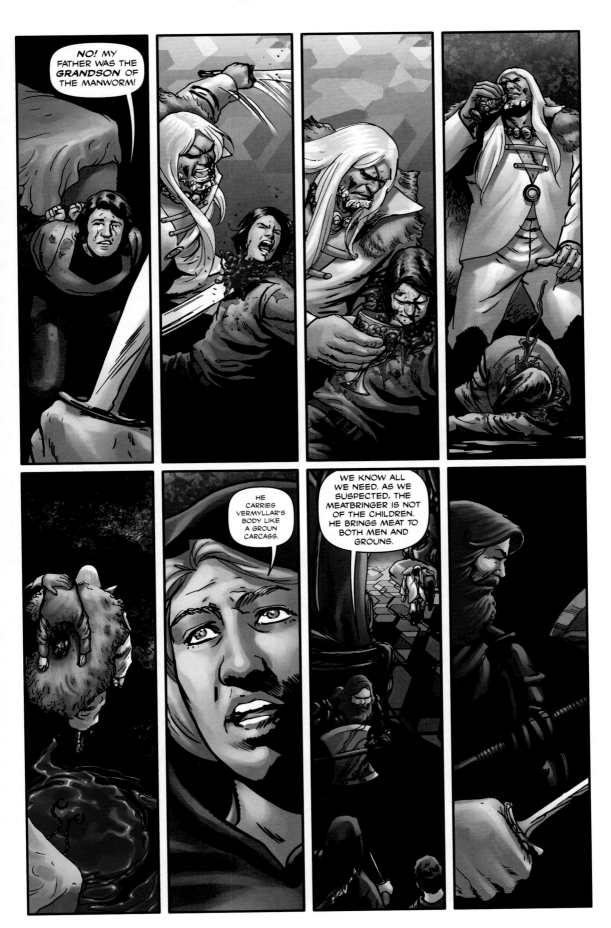

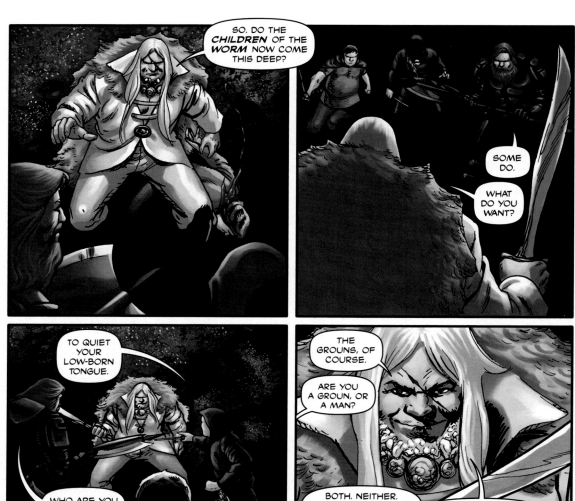

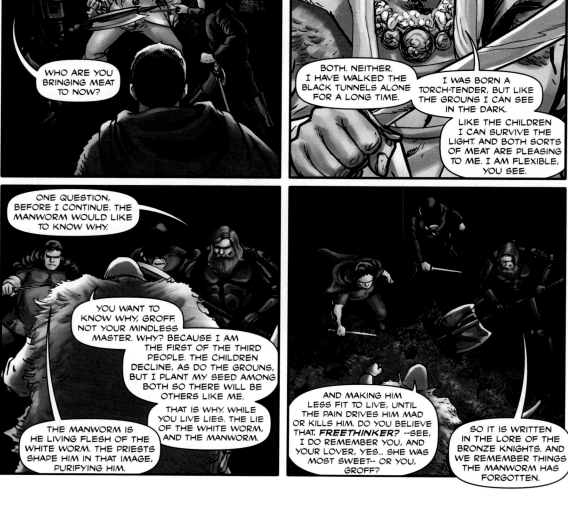

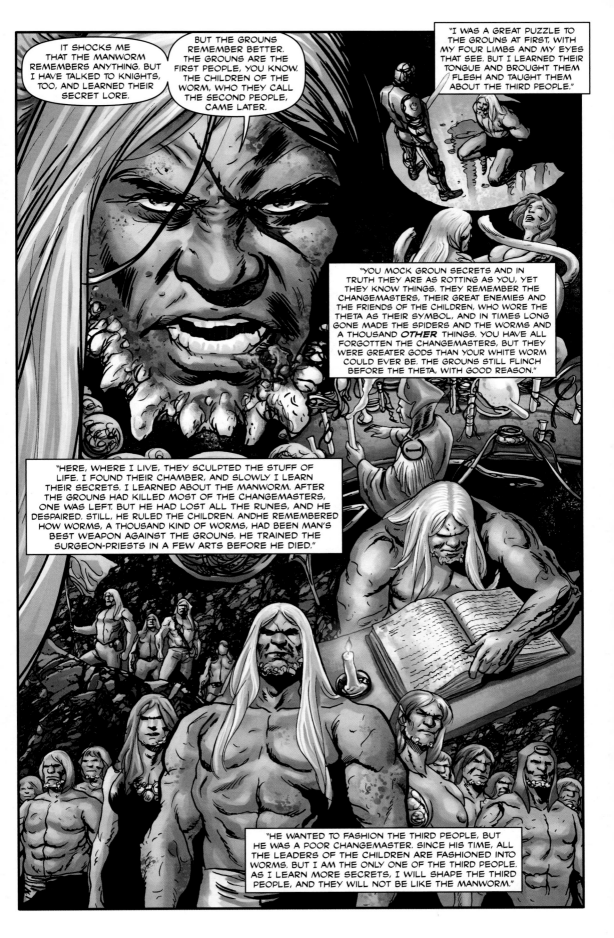

IT SHOCKS ME THAT THE MANWORM REMEMBERS ANYTHING. BUT I HAVE TALKED TO KNIGHTS, TOO, AND LEARNED THEIR SECRET LORE.

BUT THE GROUNS REMEMBER BETTER. THE GROUNS ARE THE FIRST PEOPLE, YOU KNOW. THE CHILDREN OF THE WORM, WHO THEY CALL THE SECOND PEOPLE, CAME LATER.

"I WAS A GREAT PUZZLE TO THE GROUNS AT FIRST, WITH MY FOUR LIMBS AND MY EYES THAT SEE. BUT I LEARNED THEIR TONGUE AND BROUGHT THEM FLESH AND TAUGHT THEM ABOUT THE THIRD PEOPLE."

"YOU MOCK GROUN SECRETS AND IN TRUTH THEY ARE AS ROTTING AS YOU, YET THEY KNOW THINGS. THEY REMEMBER THE CHANGEMASTERS, THEIR GREAT ENEMIES AND THE FRIENDS OF THE CHILDREN, WHO WORE THE THETA AS THEIR SYMBOL, AND IN TIMES LONG GONE MADE THE SPIDERS AND THE WORMS AND A THOUSAND *OTHER* THINGS. YOU HAVE ALL FORGOTTEN THE CHANGEMASTERS, BUT THEY WERE GREATER GODS THAN YOUR WHITE WORM COULD EVER BE. THE GROUNS STILL FLINCH BEFORE THE THETA, WITH GOOD REASON."

"HERE, WHERE I LIVE, THEY SCULPTED THE STUFF OF LIFE. I FOUND THEIR CHAMBER, AND SLOWLY I LEARN THEIR SECRETS. I LEARNED ABOUT THE MANWORM. AFTER THE GROUNS HAD KILLED MOST OF THE CHANGEMASTERS, ONE WAS LEFT. BUT HE HAD LOST ALL THE RUNES, AND HE DESPAIRED. STILL, HE RULED THE CHILDREN. ANDHE REMEMBERED HOW WORMS, A THOUSAND KIND OF WORMS, HAD BEEN MAN'S BEST WEAPON AGAINST THE GROUNS. HE TRAINED THE SURGEON-PRIESTS IN A FEW ARTS BEFORE HE DIED."

"HE WANTED TO FASHION THE THIRD PEOPLE, BUT HE WAS A POOR CHANGEMASTER. SINCE HIS TIME, ALL THE LEADERS OF THE CHILDREN ARE FASHIONED INTO WORMS. BUT I AM THE ONLY ONE OF THE THIRD PEOPLE. AS I LEARN MORE SECRETS, I WILL SHAPE THE THIRD PEOPLE, AND THEY WILL NOT BE LIKE THE MANWORM."

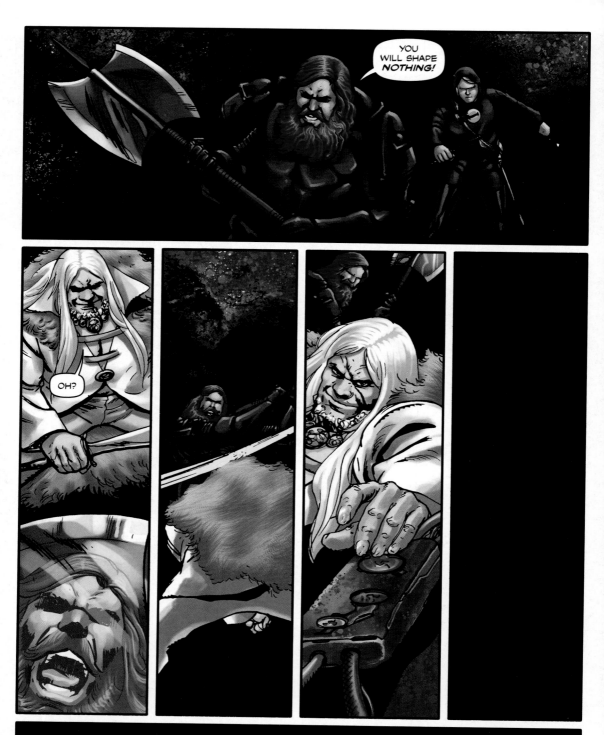

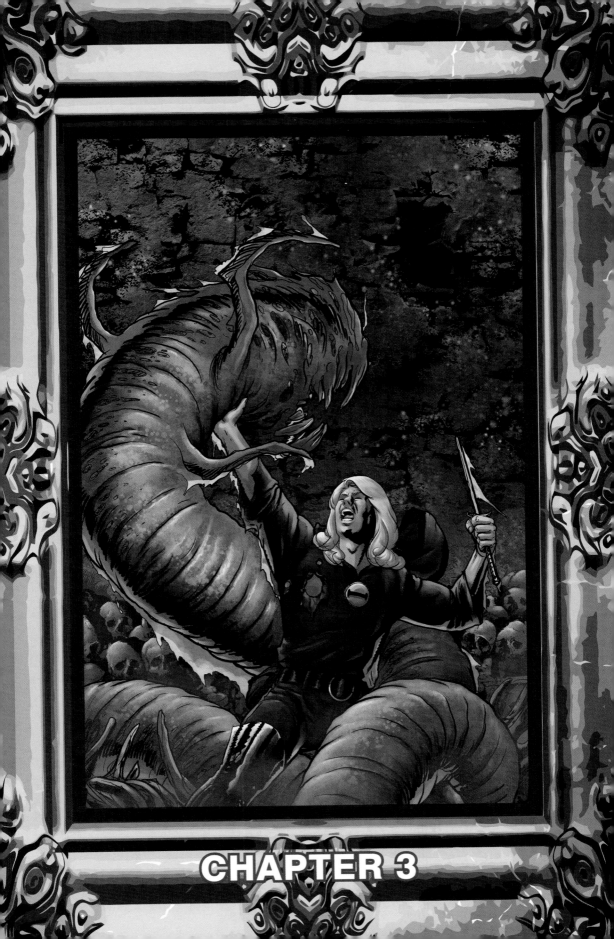

CHAPTER 3

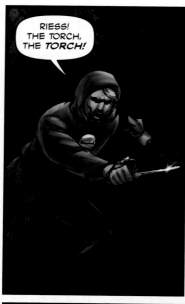

RIESS! THE TORCH, THE *TORCH!*

SSSWWIIIIISSHHH!

CLLLAANNGGG!

AAAEEIIIIIIII!

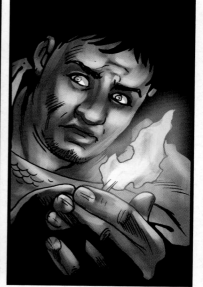

AYYYYYYY!

HAHAHAHA!

RIESS IS DEAD AND GROFF I DON'T KNOW AND THE MEATBRINGER LAUGHING...

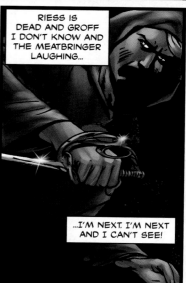

...I'M NEXT. I'M NEXT AND I CAN'T SEE!

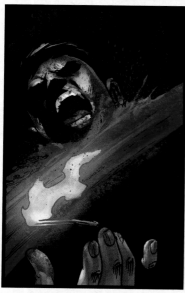

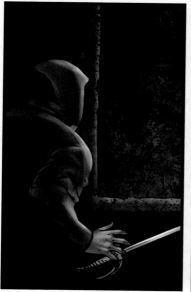

THE ROPE, THE ROPE, WHERE *IS* IT...?

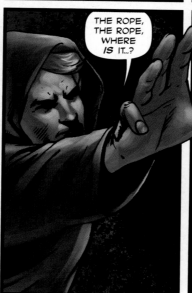

THWWACKKK! THWWACKKK!

OHHH -UHHHHHH...

...THE MEATBRINGER IS CHOPPING HIS MEAT... AHHH...

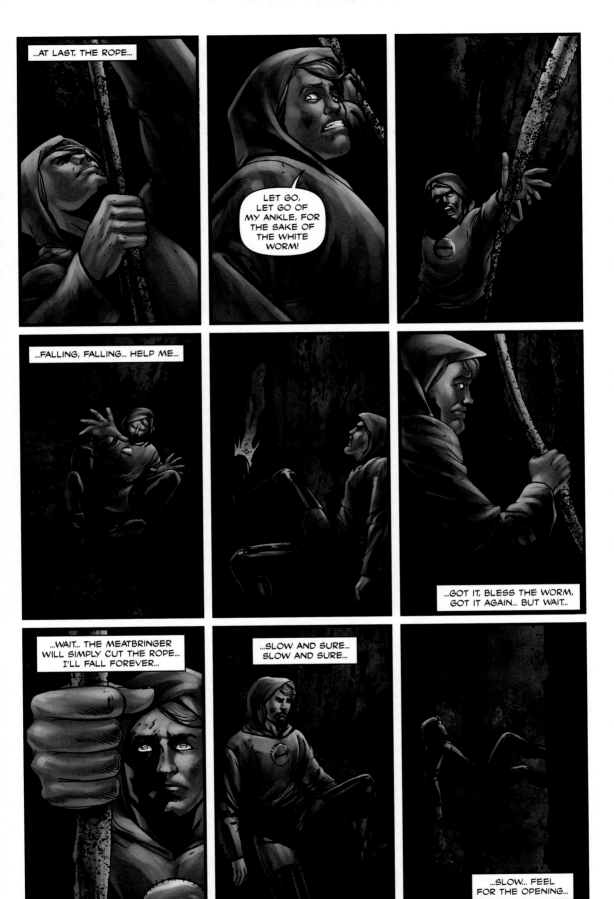

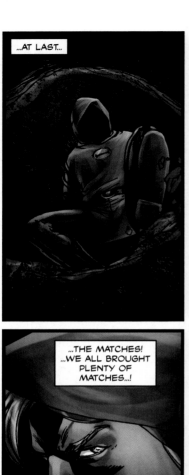

...AT LAST...

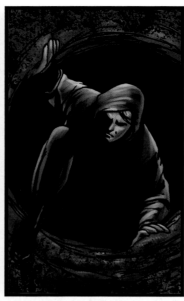

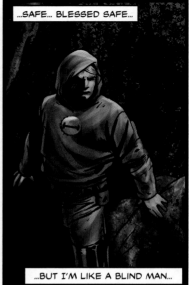

...SAFE... BLESSED SAFE...

...BUT I'M LIKE A BLIND MAN...

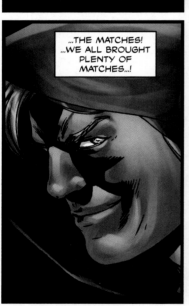

...THE MATCHES! ...WE ALL BROUGHT PLENTY OF MATCHES...!

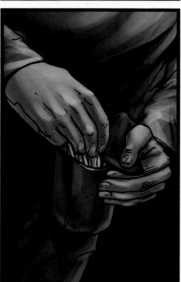

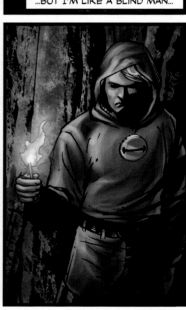

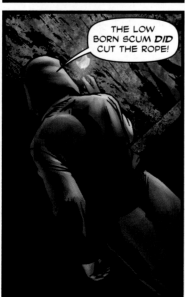

THE LOW BORN SCUM *DID* CUT THE ROPE!

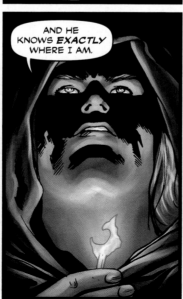

AND HE KNOWS *EXACTLY* WHERE I AM.

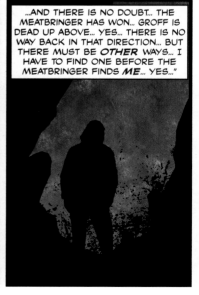

...AND THERE IS NO DOUBT... THE MEATBRINGER HAS WON... GROFF IS DEAD UP ABOVE... YES... THERE IS NO WAY BACK IN THAT DIRECTION... BUT THERE MUST BE *OTHER* WAYS... I HAVE TO FIND ONE BEFORE THE MEATBRINGER FINDS *ME*... YES..."

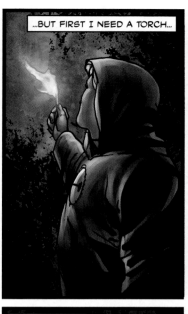

...BUT FIRST I NEED A TORCH...

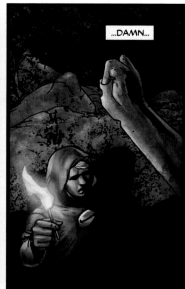

...DAMN...

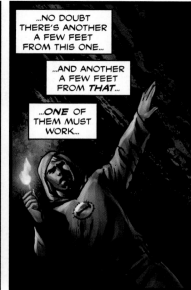

...NO DOUBT THERE'S ANOTHER A FEW FEET FROM THIS ONE...

...AND ANOTHER A FEW FEET FROM *THAT*...

...*ONE* OF THEM MUST WORK...

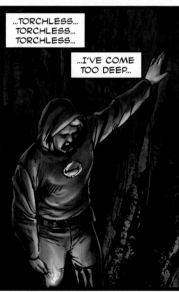

...TORCHLESS... TORCHLESS... TORCHLESS...

...I'VE COME TOO DEEP...

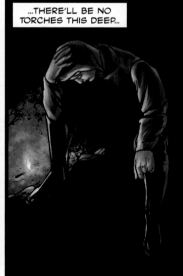

...THERE'LL BE NO TORCHES THIS DEEP...

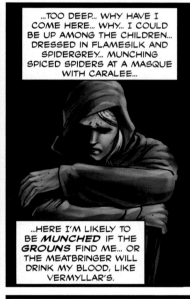

...TOO DEEP... WHY HAVE I COME HERE... WHY... I COULD BE UP AMONG THE CHILDREN... DRESSED IN FLAMESILK AND SPIDERGREY... MUNCHING SPICED SPIDERS AT A MASQUE WITH CARALEE...

...HERE I'M LIKELY TO BE *MUNCHED* IF THE *GROUNS* FIND ME... OR THE MEATBRINGER WILL DRINK MY BLOOD, LIKE VERMYLLAR'S.

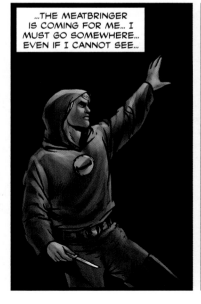

...THE MEATBRINGER IS COMING FOR ME... I MUST GO SOMEWHERE... EVEN IF I CANNOT SEE...

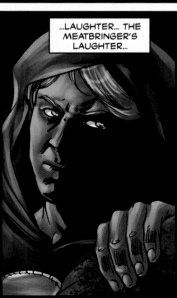

...LAUGHTER... THE MEATBRINGER'S LAUGHTER...

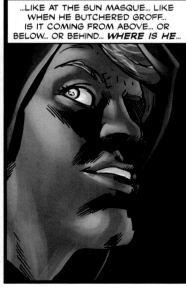

...LIKE AT THE SUN MASQUE... LIKE WHEN HE BUTCHERED GROFF... IS IT COMING FROM ABOVE... OR BELOW... OR BEHIND... *WHERE IS HE*...

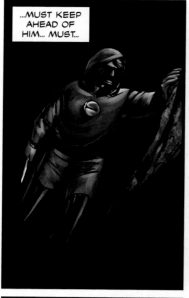

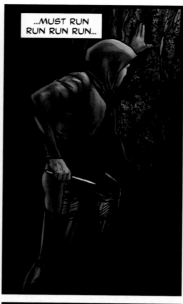

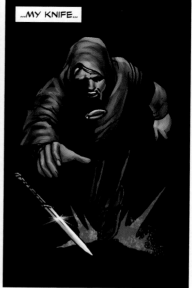

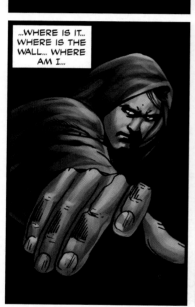

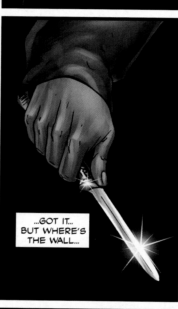

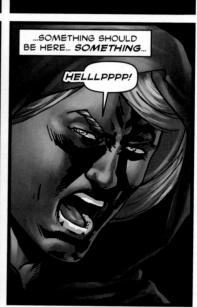

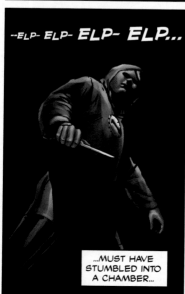

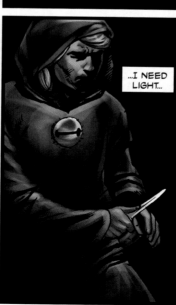

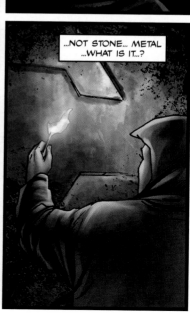

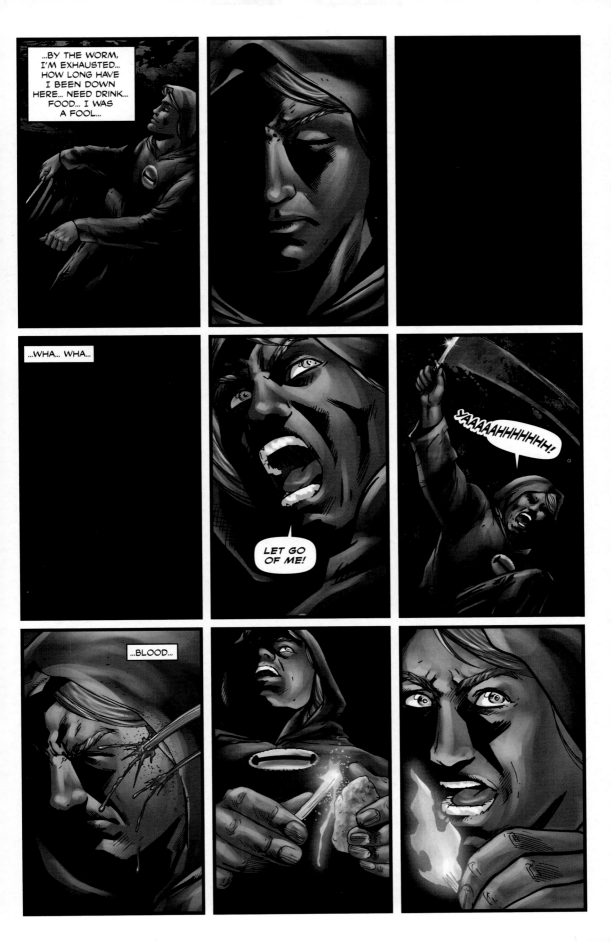

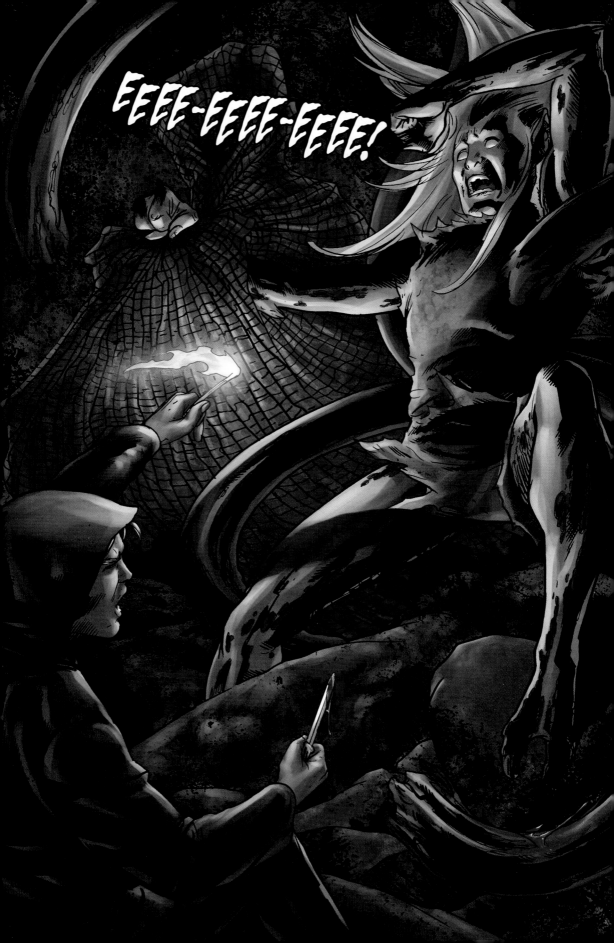

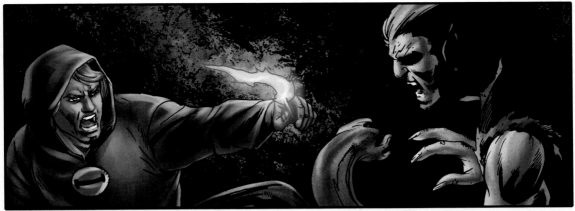

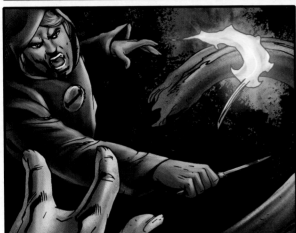

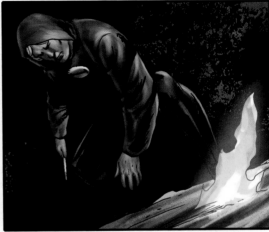

...CIRCLING FROM BEHIND...

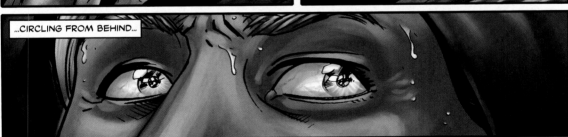

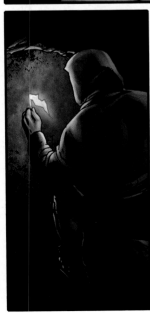

...QUIET... QUIET...
STAB THE THING...

...SOFT, PADDED,
SNEAKING,
SILENT FEET...

...CAN'T FIGHT
IT WITHOUT A
TORCH... WITHOUT
LIGHT TO SEE BY...

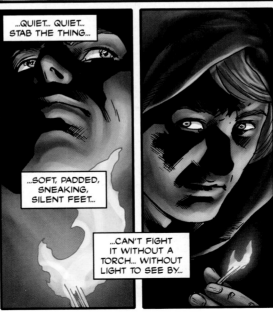

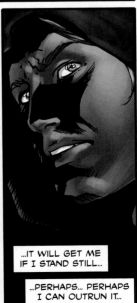

...IT WILL GET ME
IF I STAND STILL...

...PERHAPS... PERHAPS
I CAN OUTRUN IT...

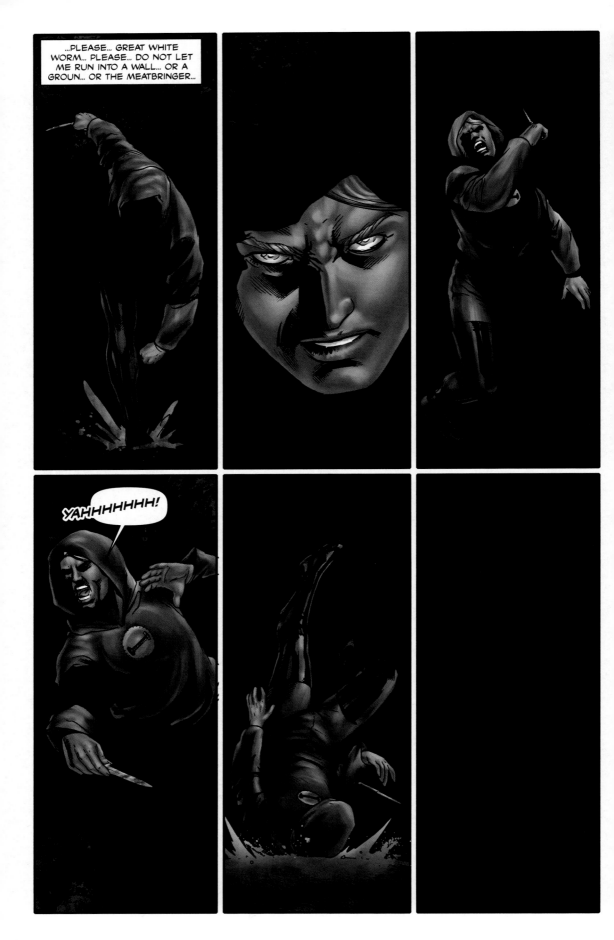

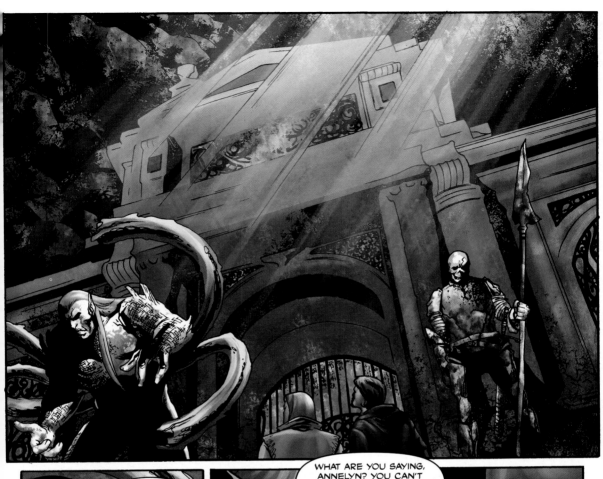

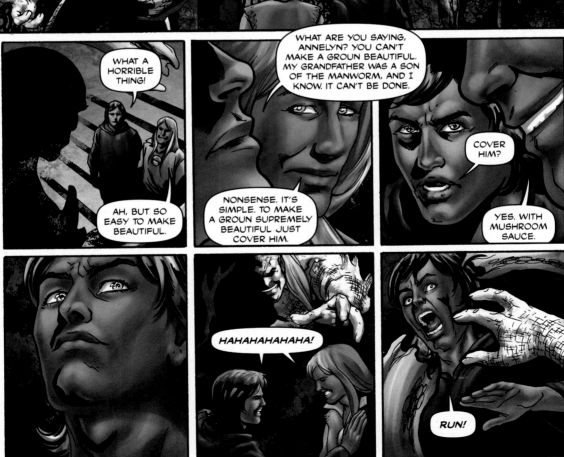

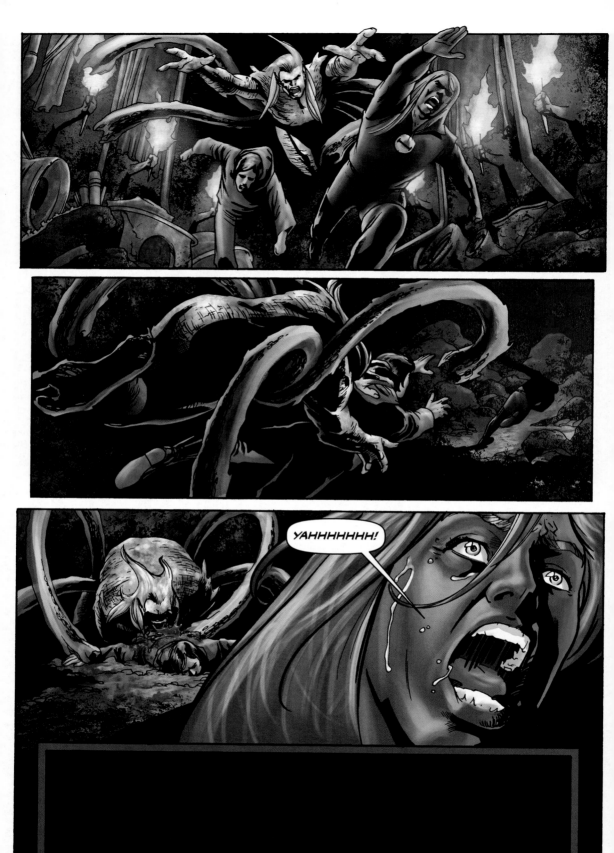

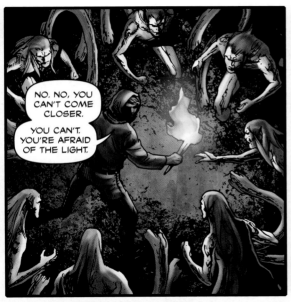

NO, NO, YOU CAN'T COME CLOSER.

YOU CAN'T. YOU'RE AFRAID OF THE LIGHT.

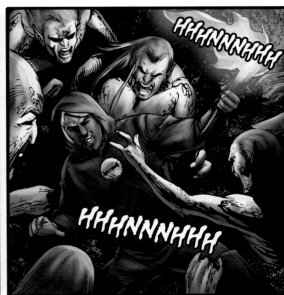

HHHNNNHHH

HHHNNNHHH

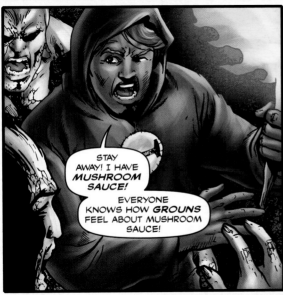

STAY AWAY! I HAVE *MUSHROOM SAUCE!*

EVERYONE KNOWS HOW *GROUNS* FEEL ABOUT MUSHROOM SAUCE!

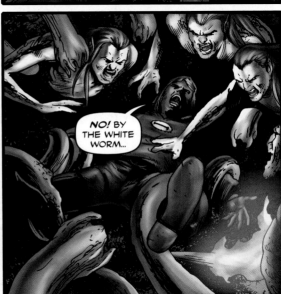

NO! BY THE WHITE WORM...

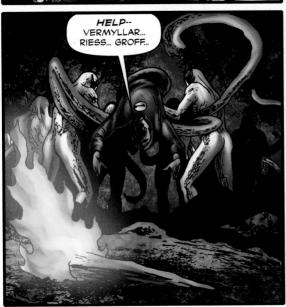

HELP-- VERMYLLAR... RIESS... GROFF...

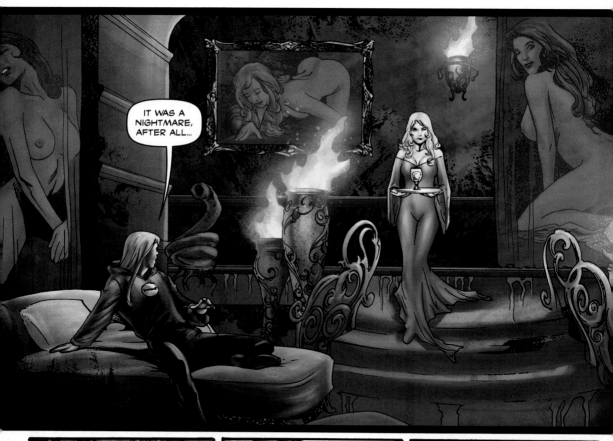

IT WAS A NIGHTMARE, AFTER ALL...

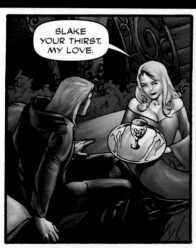

SLAKE YOUR THIRST, MY LOVE.

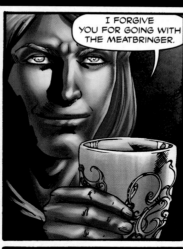

I FORGIVE YOU FOR GOING WITH THE MEATBRINGER.

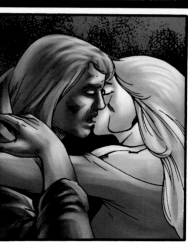

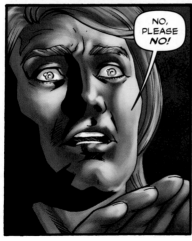

NO, PLEASE NO!

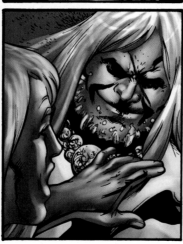

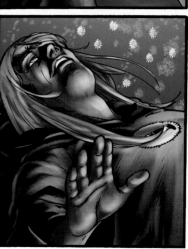

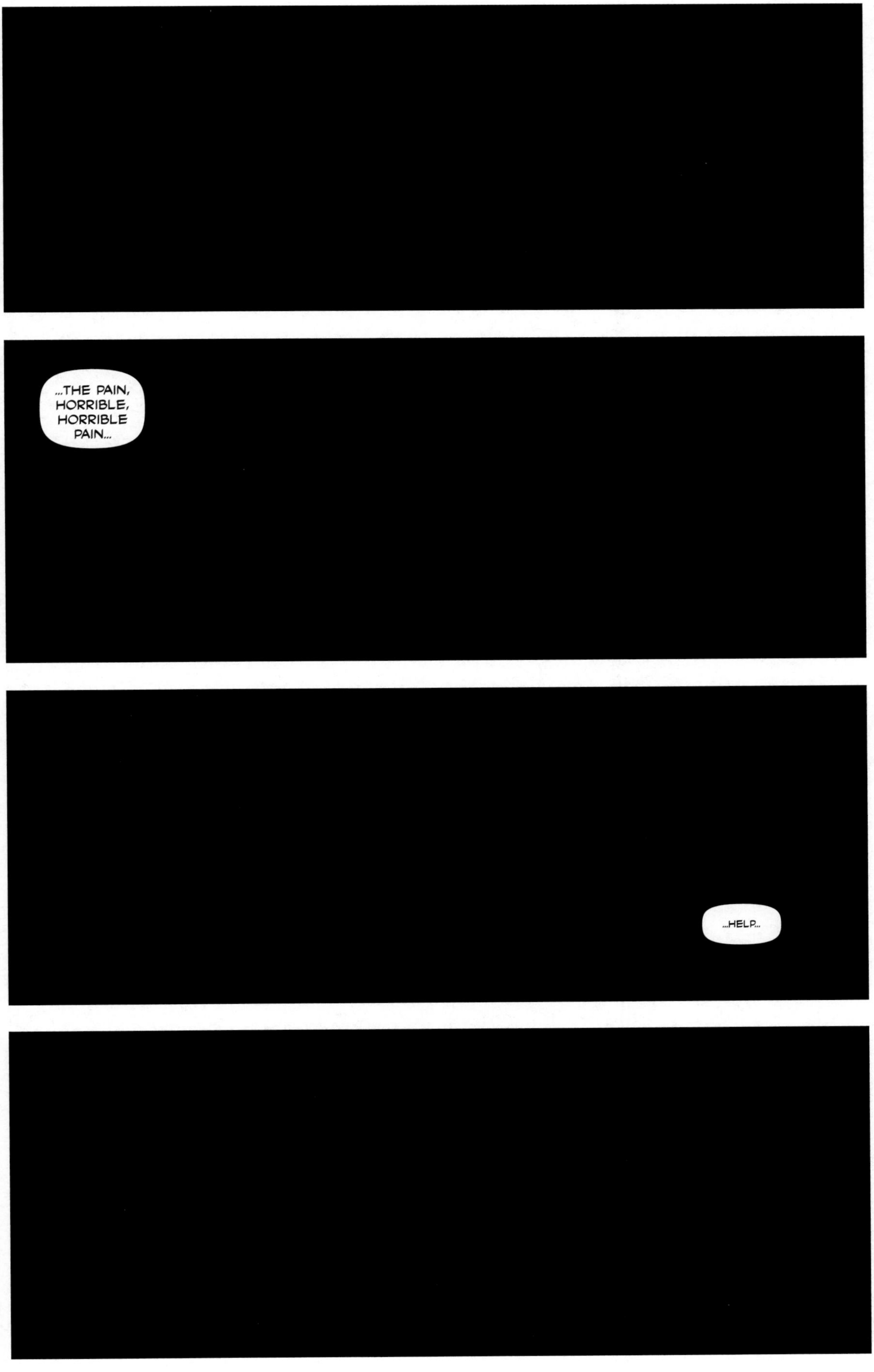
...THE PAIN, HORRIBLE, HORRIBLE PAIN...
...HELP...

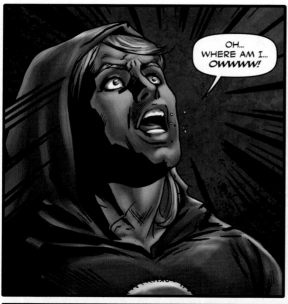

OH... WHERE AM I... OWWWW!

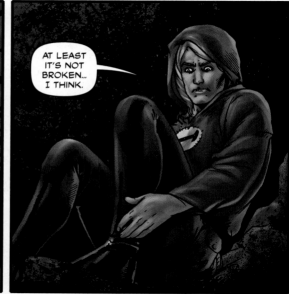

AT LEAST IT'S NOT BROKEN... I THINK.

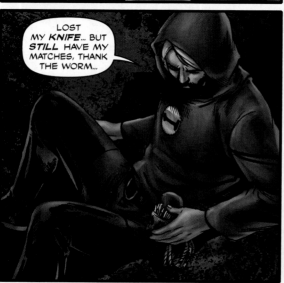

LOST MY *KNIFE*... BUT *STILL* HAVE MY MATCHES, THANK THE WORM...

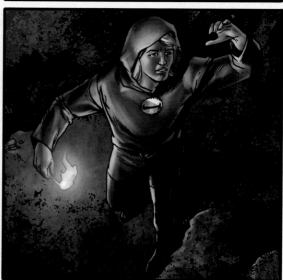

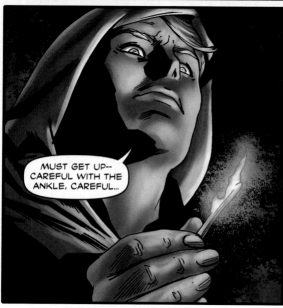

MUST GET UP-- CAREFUL WITH THE ANKLE, CAREFUL...

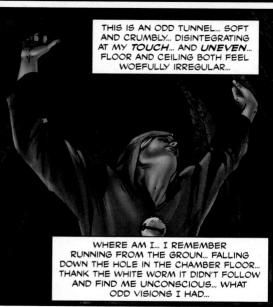

THIS IS AN ODD TUNNEL... SOFT AND CRUMBLY... DISINTEGRATING AT MY *TOUCH*... AND *UNEVEN*... FLOOR AND CEILING BOTH FEEL WOEFULLY IRREGULAR...

WHERE AM I... I REMEMBER RUNNING FROM THE GROUN... FALLING DOWN THE HOLE IN THE CHAMBER FLOOR... THANK THE WHITE WORM IT DIDN'T FOLLOW AND FIND ME UNCONSCIOUS... WHAT ODD VISIONS I HAD...

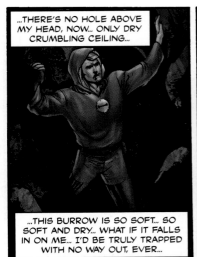

...THERE'S NO HOLE ABOVE MY HEAD, NOW... ONLY DRY CRUMBLING CEILING...

...THIS BURROW IS SO SOFT... SO SOFT AND DRY... WHAT IF IT FALLS IN ON ME... I'D BE TRULY TRAPPED WITH NO WAY OUT, EVER...

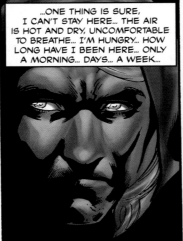

...ONE THING IS SURE, I CAN'T STAY HERE... THE AIR IS HOT AND DRY, UNCOMFORTABLE TO BREATHE... I'M HUNGRY... HOW LONG HAVE I BEEN HERE... ONLY A MORNING... DAYS... A WEEK...

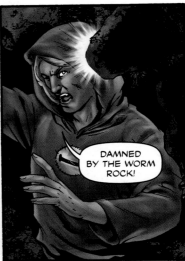

DAMNED BY THE WORM ROCK!

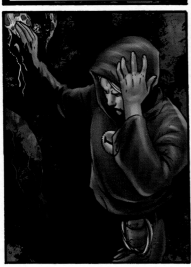

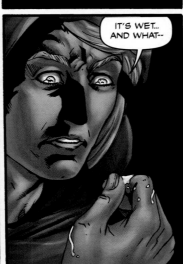

IT'S WET... AND WHAT--

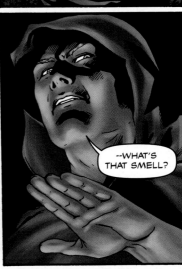

--WHAT'S THAT SMELL?

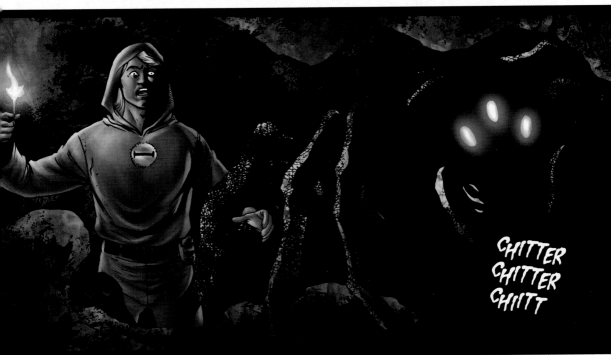

CHITTER CHITTER CHIITT

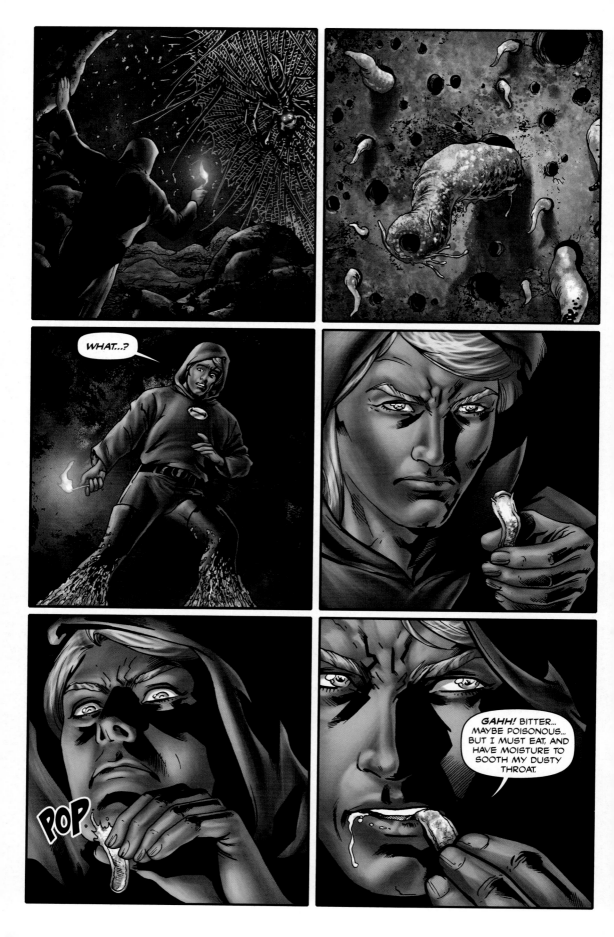

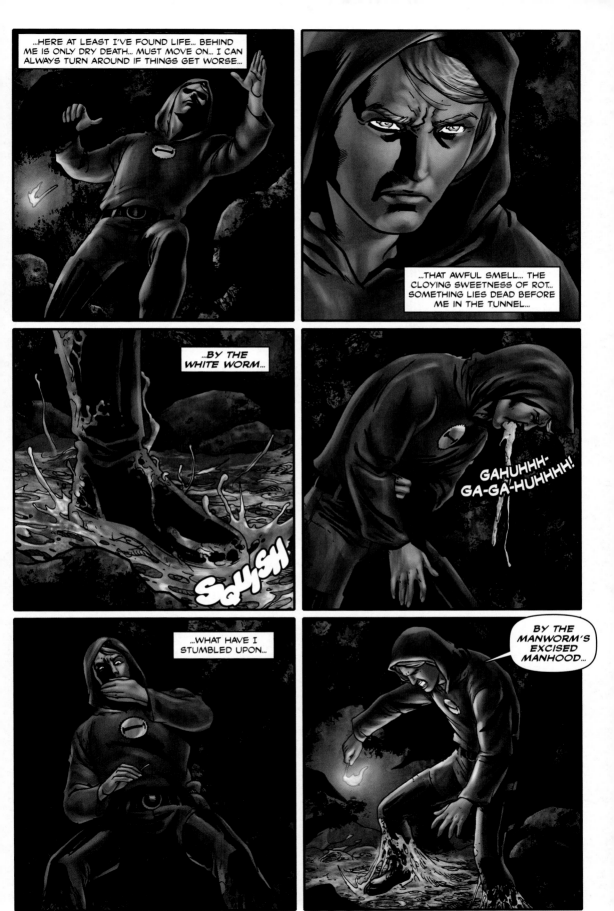

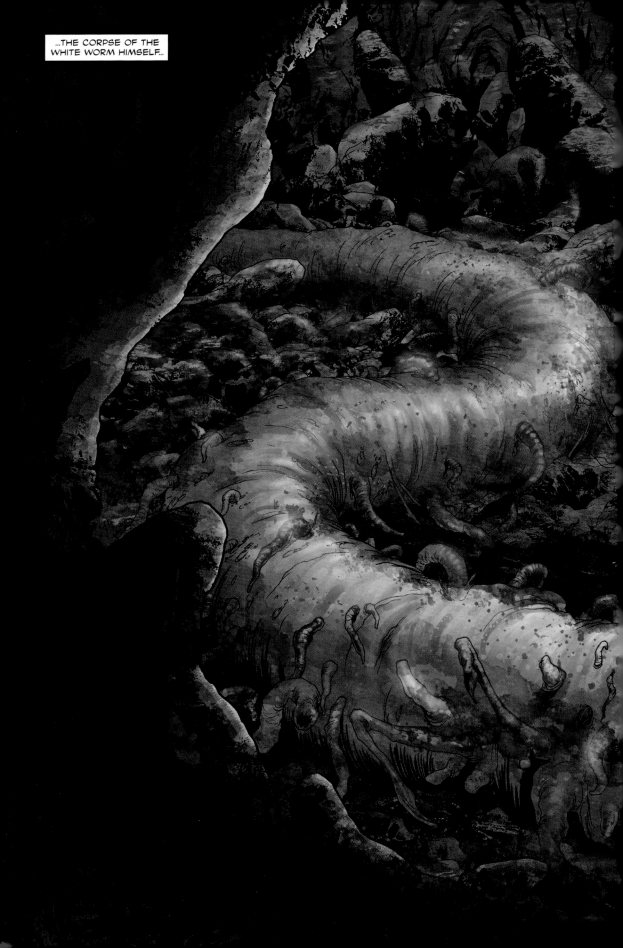

...THE CORPSE OF THE WHITE WORM HIMSELF...

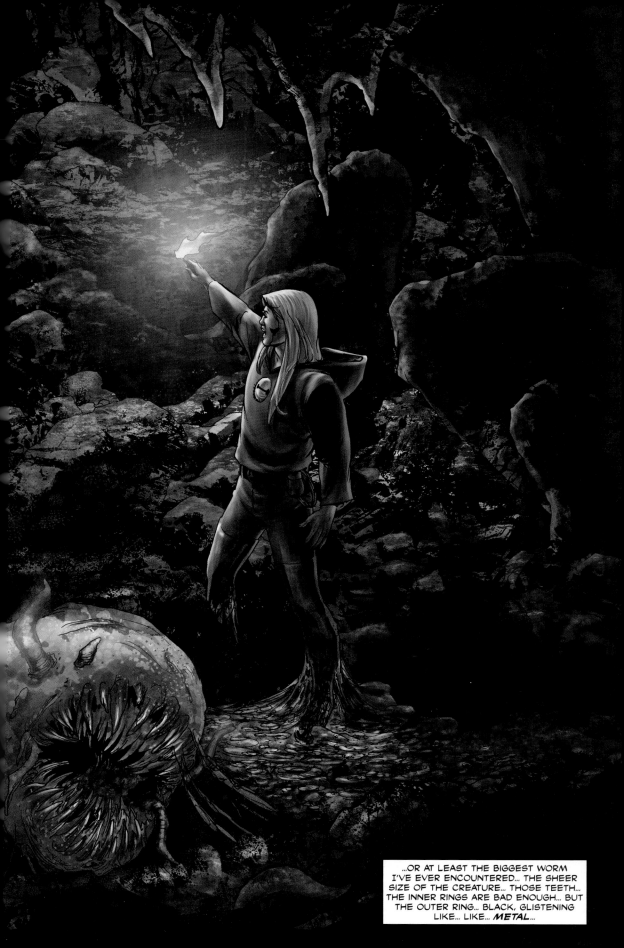

...OR AT LEAST THE BIGGEST WORM
I'VE EVER ENCOUNTERED... THE SHEER
SIZE OF THE CREATURE... THOSE TEETH...
THE INNER RINGS ARE BAD ENOUGH... BUT
THE OUTER RING... BLACK, GLISTENING
LIKE... LIKE... *METAL*...

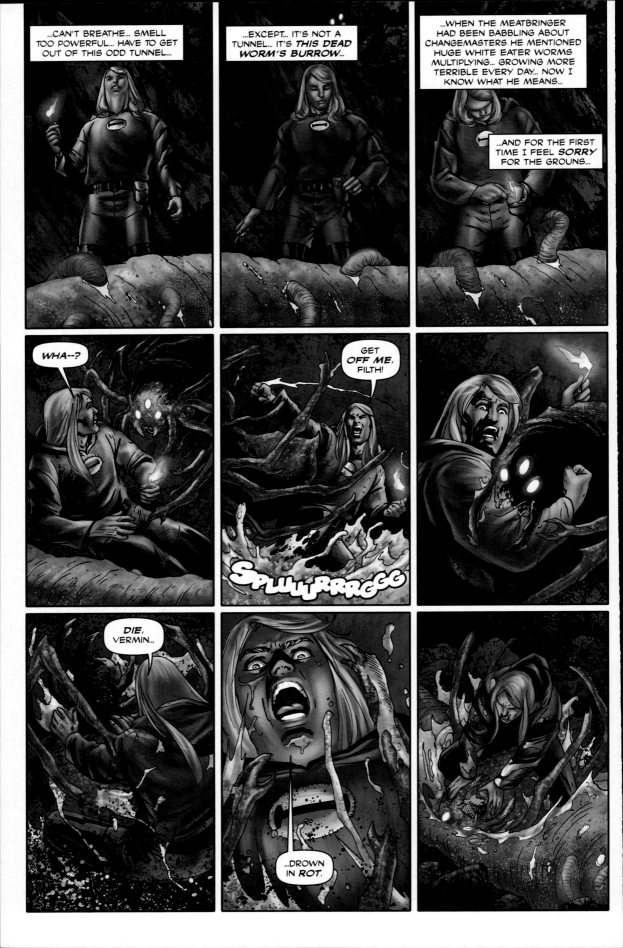

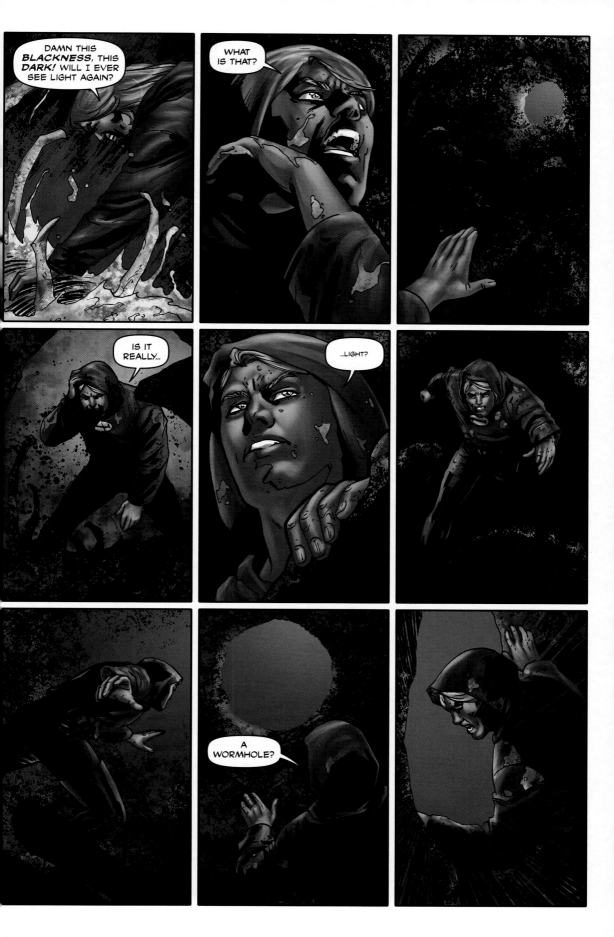

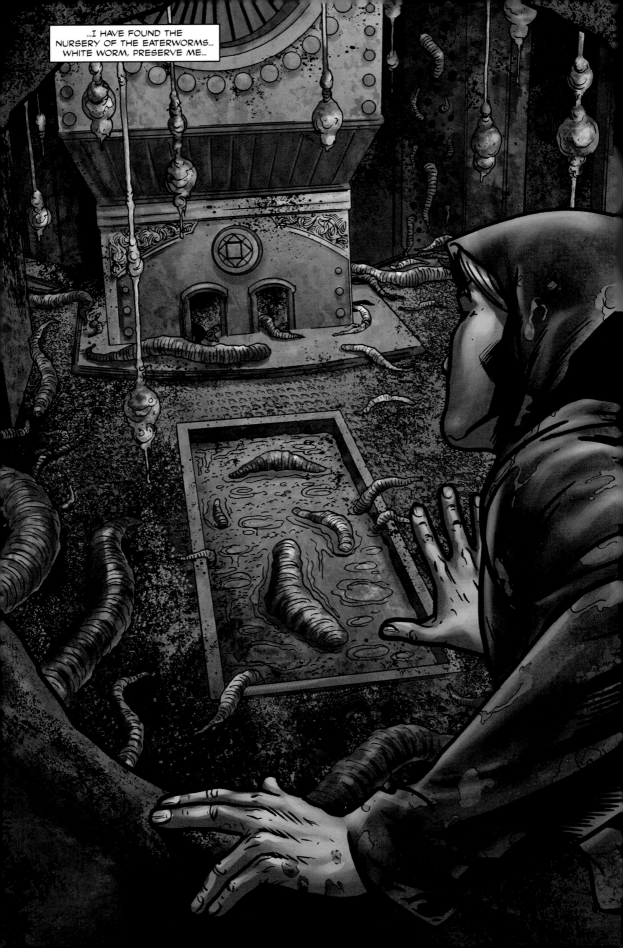

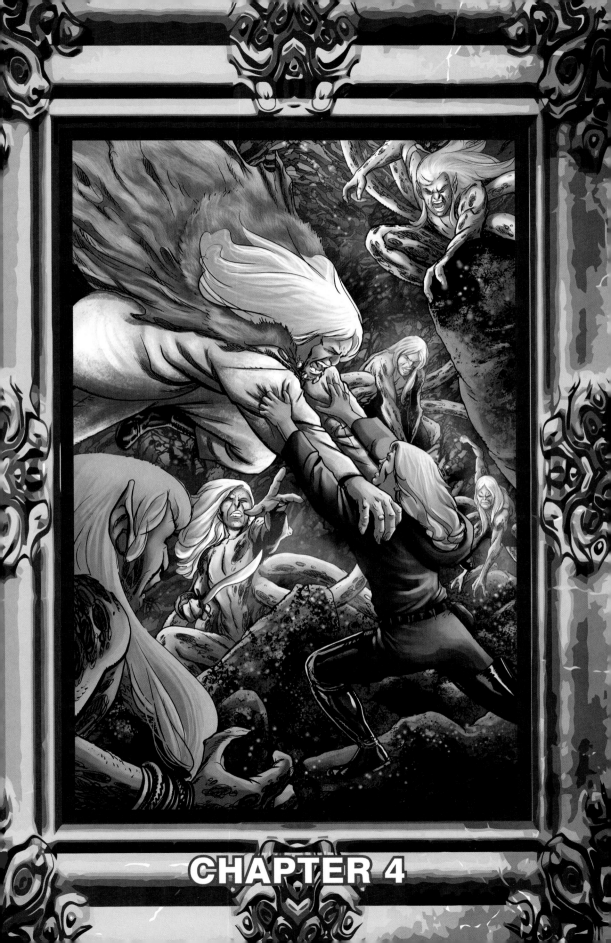

CHAPTER 4

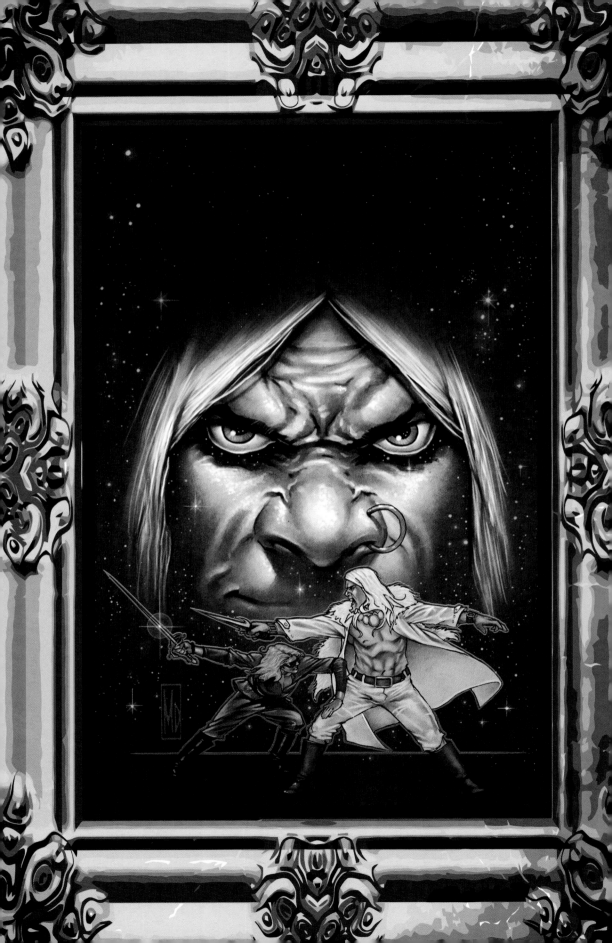

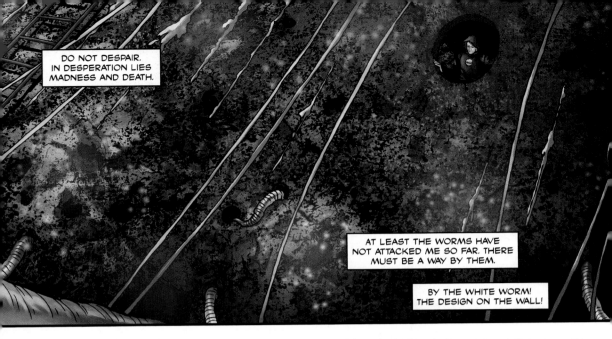

DO NOT DESPAIR. IN DESPERATION LIES MADNESS AND DEATH.

AT LEAST THE WORMS HAVE NOT ATTACKED ME SO FAR. THERE MUST BE A WAY BY THEM.

BY THE WHITE WORM! THE DESIGN ON THE WALL!

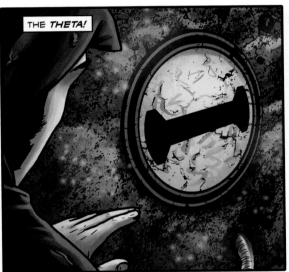

THE *THETA!*

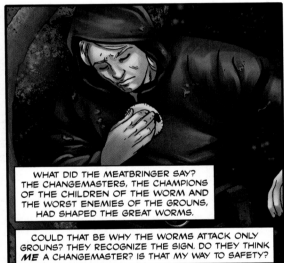

WHAT DID THE MEATBRINGER SAY? THE CHANGEMASTERS, THE CHAMPIONS OF THE CHILDREN OF THE WORM AND THE WORST ENEMIES OF THE GROUNS, HAD SHAPED THE GREAT WORMS.

COULD THAT BE WHY THE WORMS ATTACK ONLY GROUNS? THEY RECOGNIZE THE SIGN. DO THEY THINK *ME* A CHANGEMASTER? IS THAT MY WAY TO SAFETY?

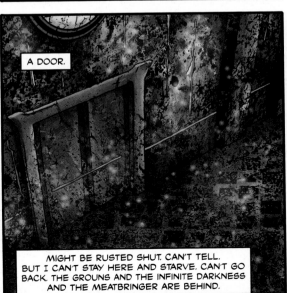

A DOOR.

MIGHT BE RUSTED SHUT. CAN'T TELL. BUT I CAN'T STAY HERE AND STARVE. CAN'T GO BACK. THE GROUNS AND THE INFINITE DARKNESS AND THE MEATBRINGER ARE BEHIND.

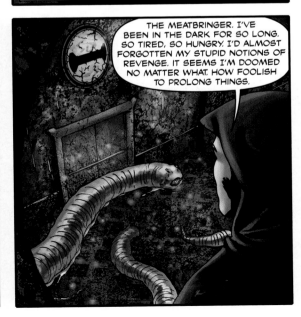

THE MEATBRINGER. I'VE BEEN IN THE DARK FOR SO LONG. SO TIRED, SO HUNGRY. I'D ALMOST FORGOTTEN MY STUPID NOTIONS OF REVENGE. IT SEEMS I'M DOOMED NO MATTER WHAT. HOW FOOLISH TO PROLONG THINGS.

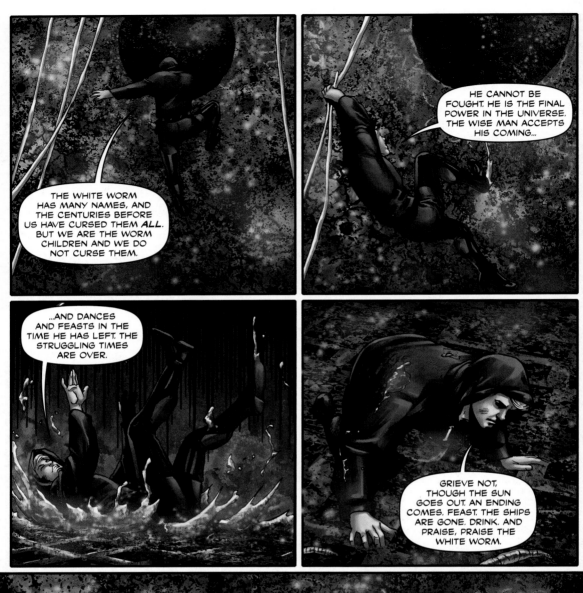

THE WHITE WORM HAS MANY NAMES, AND THE CENTURIES BEFORE US HAVE CURSED THEM *ALL*. BUT WE ARE THE WORM CHILDREN AND WE DO NOT CURSE THEM.

HE CANNOT BE FOUGHT. HE IS THE FINAL POWER IN THE UNIVERSE. THE WISE MAN ACCEPTS HIS COMING...

...AND DANCES AND FEASTS IN THE TIME HE HAS LEFT. THE STRUGGLING TIMES ARE OVER.

GRIEVE NOT, THOUGH THE SUN GOES OUT. AN ENDING COMES. FEAST. THE SHIPS ARE GONE. DRINK. AND PRAISE, PRAISE THE WHITE WORM.

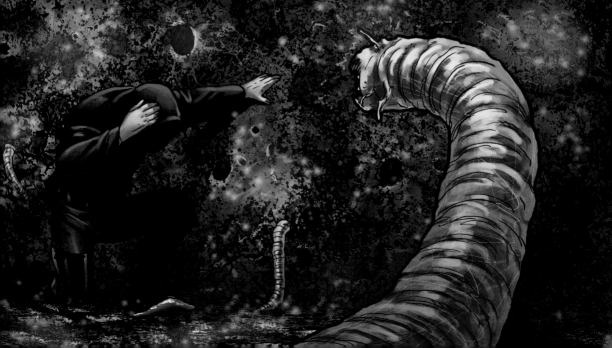

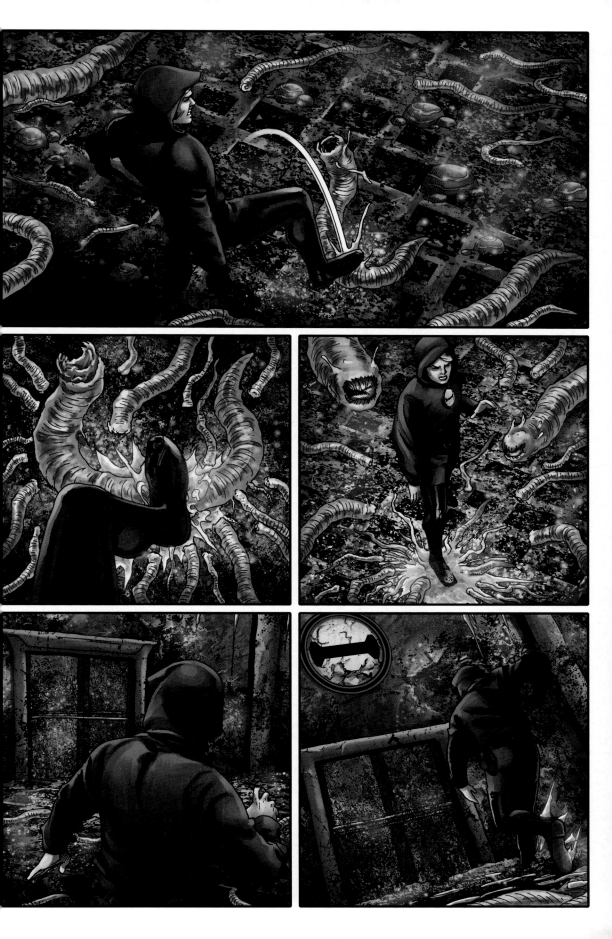

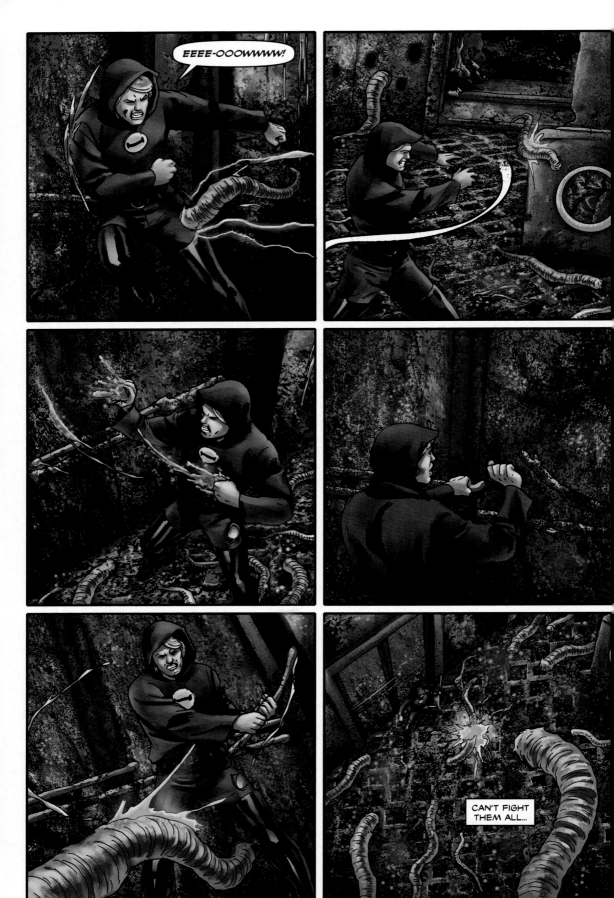

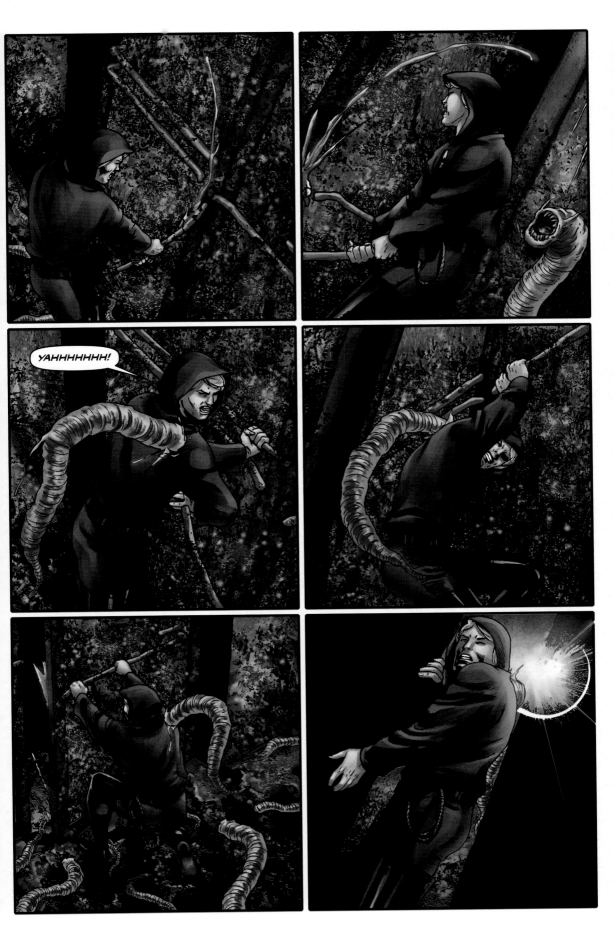

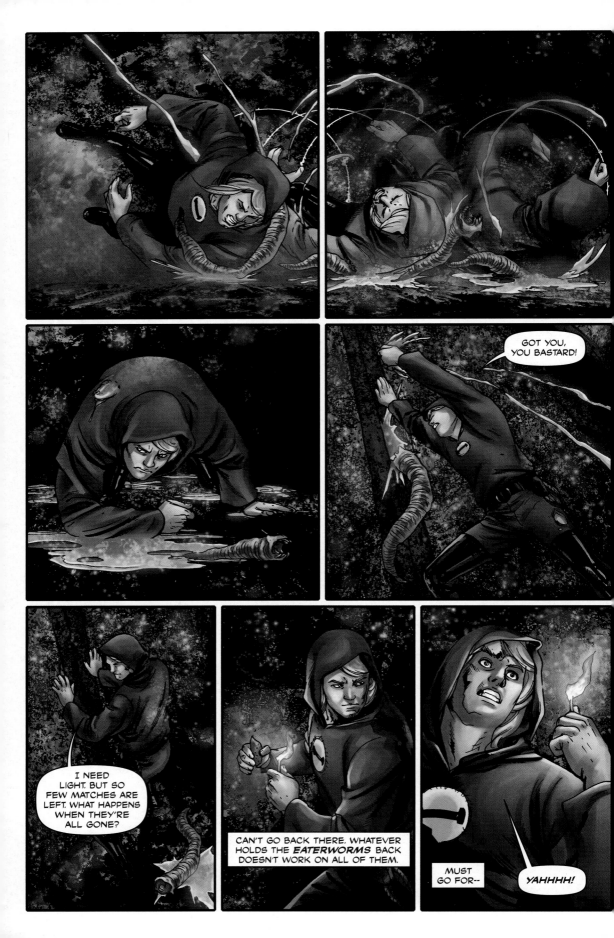

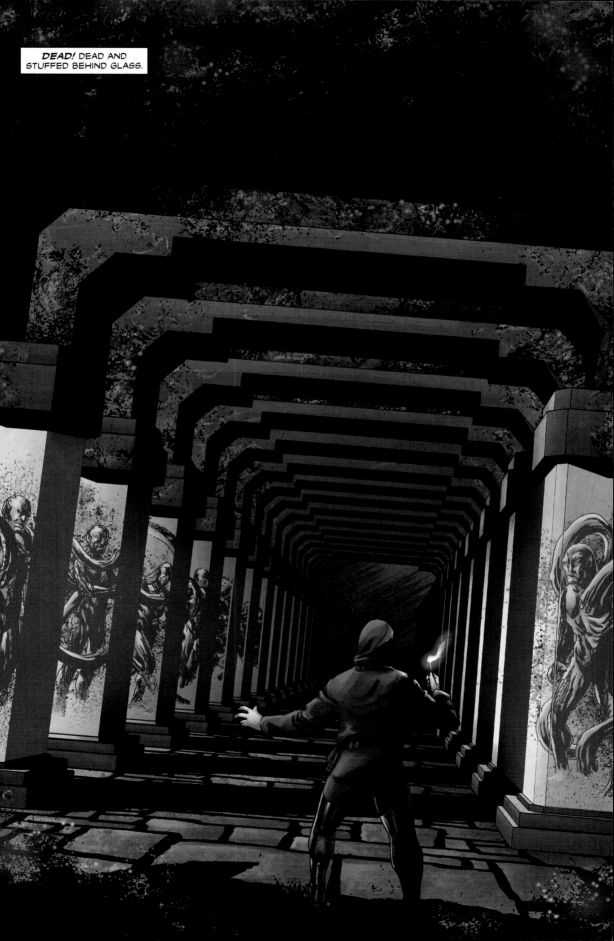

DEAD! DEAD AND STUFFED BEHIND GLASS.

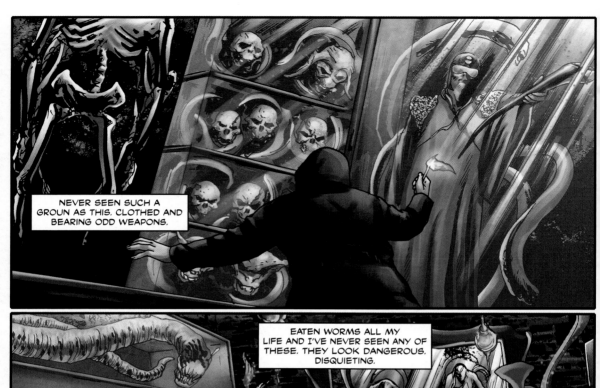

NEVER SEEN SUCH A
GROUN AS THIS. CLOTHED AND
BEARING ODD WEAPONS.

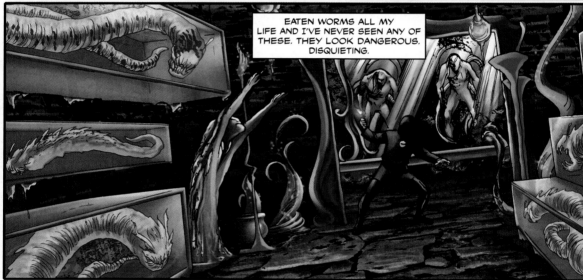

EATEN WORMS ALL MY
LIFE AND I'VE NEVER SEEN ANY OF
THESE. THEY LOOK DANGEROUS.
DISQUIETING.

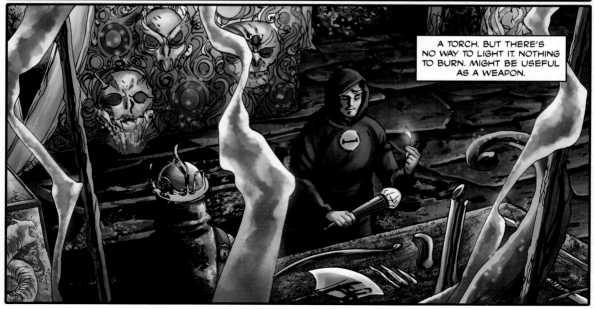

A TORCH. BUT THERE'S
NO WAY TO LIGHT IT. NOTHING
TO BURN. MIGHT BE USEFUL
AS A WEAPON.

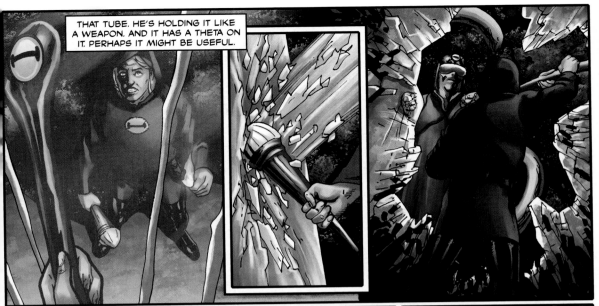

THAT TUBE. HE'S HOLDING IT LIKE A WEAPON. AND IT HAS A THETA ON IT. PERHAPS IT MIGHT BE USEFUL.

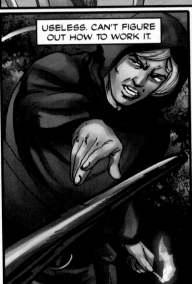

USELESS. CAN'T FIGURE OUT HOW TO WORK IT.

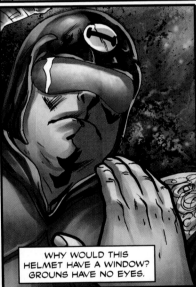

WHY WOULD THIS HELMET HAVE A WINDOW? GROUNS HAVE NO EYES.

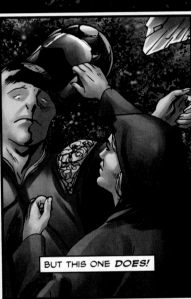

BUT THIS ONE *DOES!*

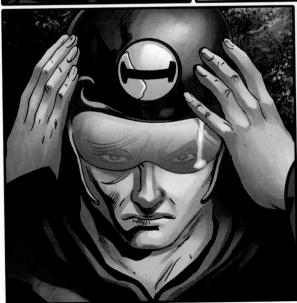

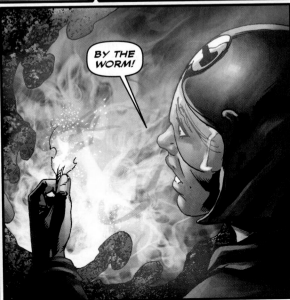

BY THE WORM!

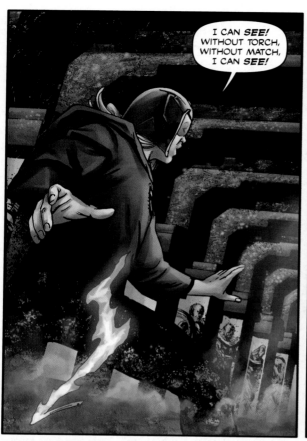

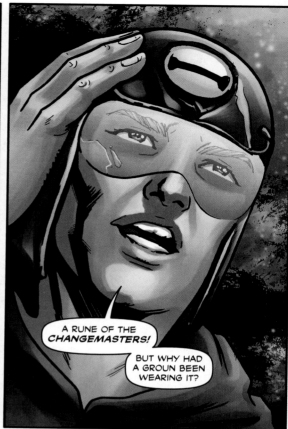

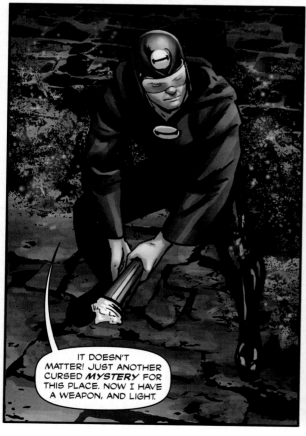

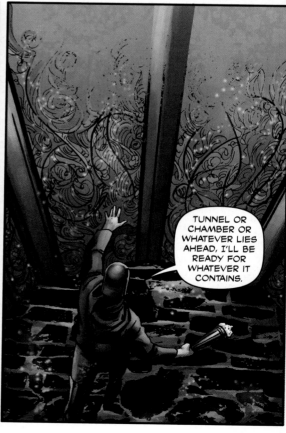

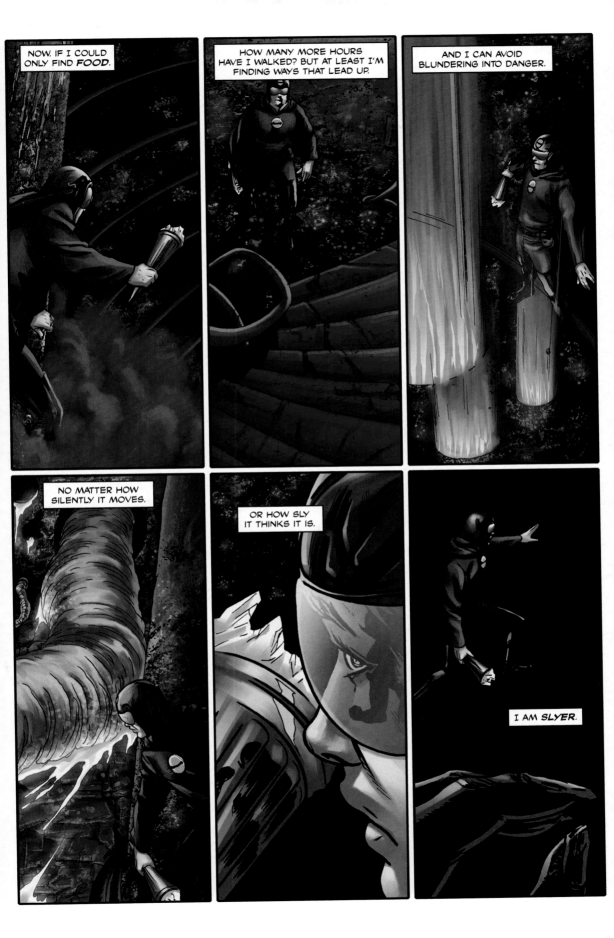

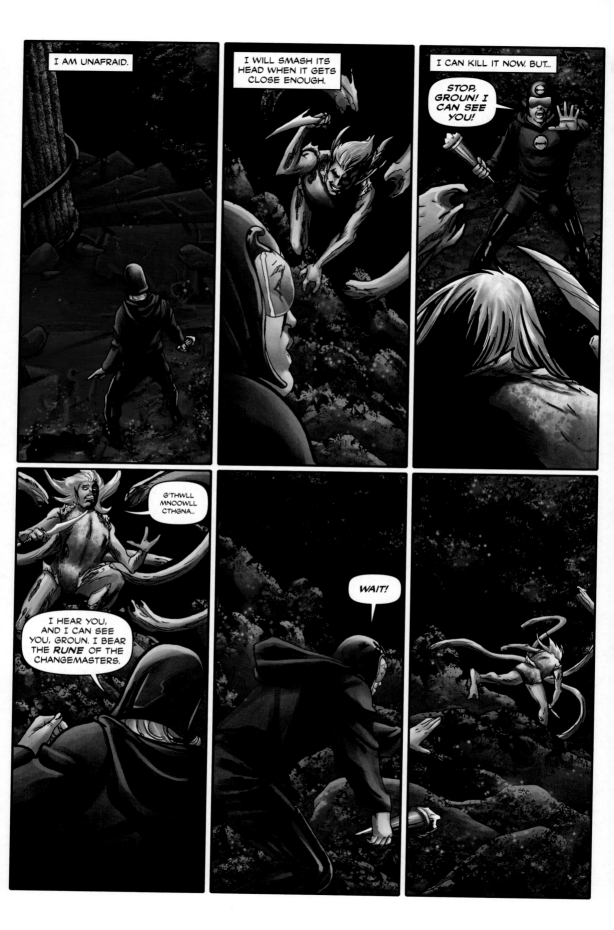

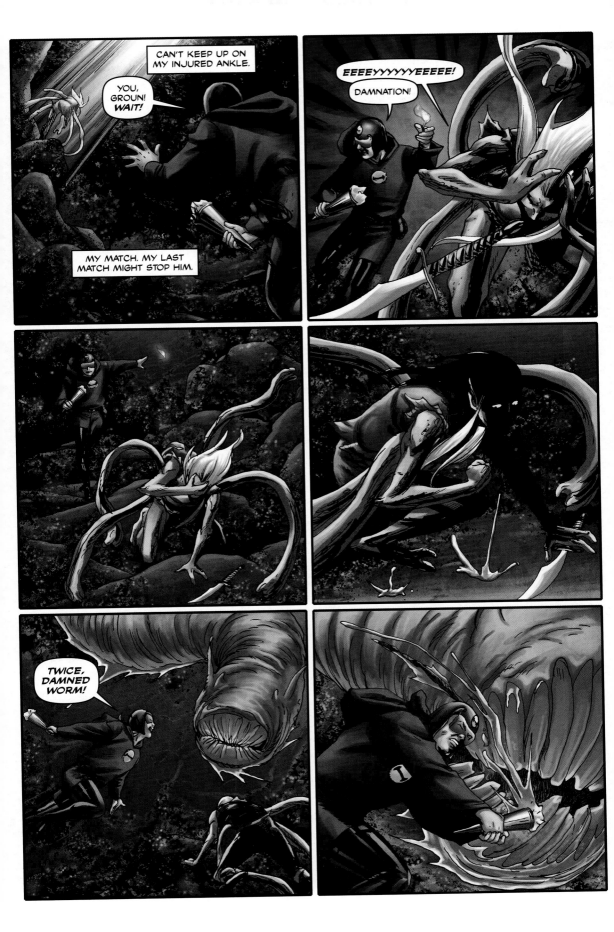

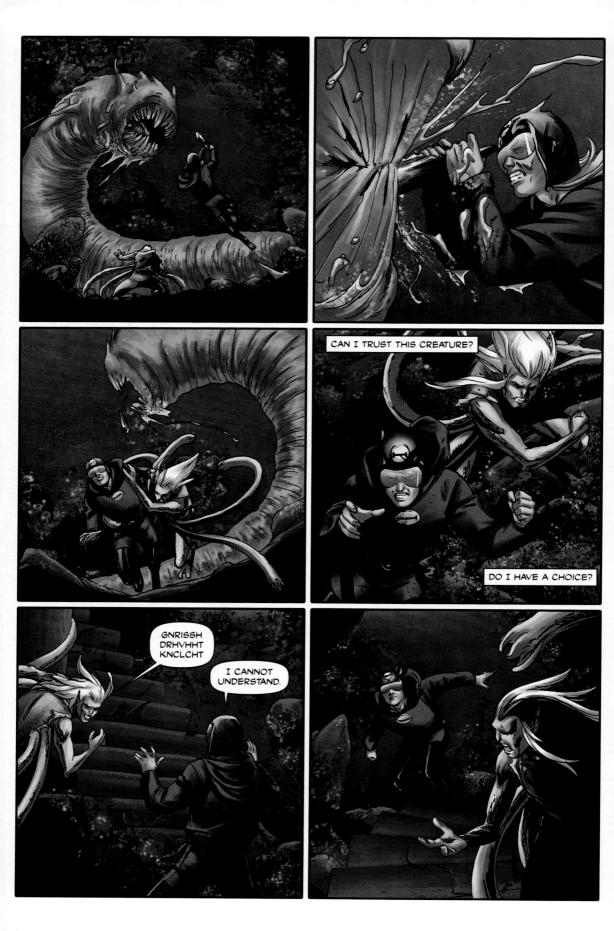

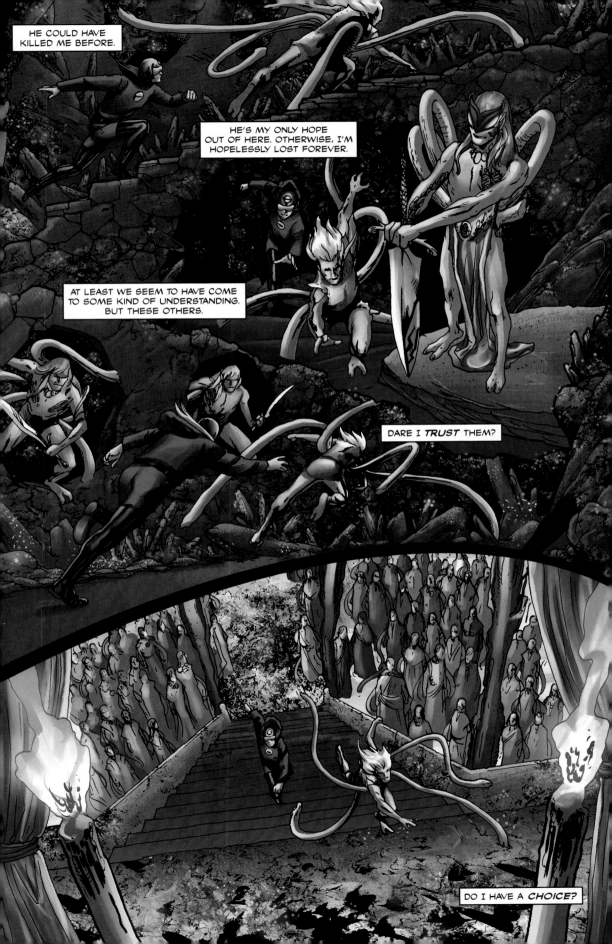

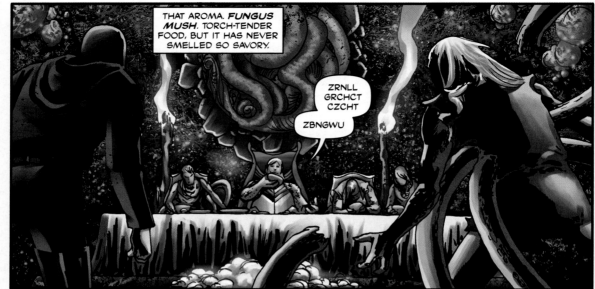

THAT AROMA. *FUNGUS MUSH.* TORCH-TENDER FOOD, BUT IT HAS NEVER SMELLED SO SAVORY.

ZRNLL GRCHCT CZCHT

ZBNGWU

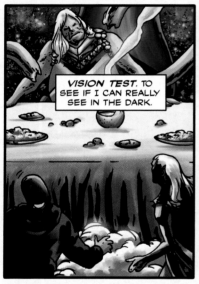

VISION TEST. TO SEE IF I CAN REALLY SEE IN THE DARK.

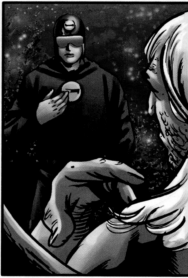

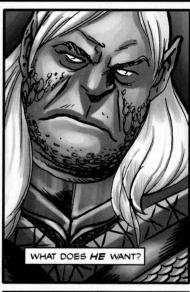

WHAT DOES *HE* WANT?

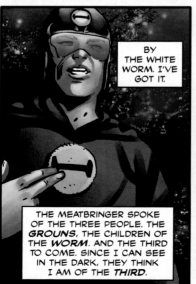

BY THE WHITE WORM. I'VE GOT IT.

THE MEATBRINGER SPOKE OF THE THREE PEOPLE. THE *GROUNS*, THE CHILDREN OF THE *WORM*. AND THE THIRD TO COME. SINCE I CAN SEE IN THE DARK, THEY THINK I AM OF THE *THIRD*.

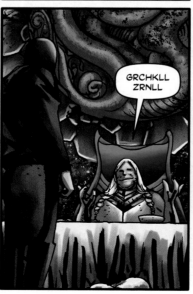

GRCHKLL ZRNLL

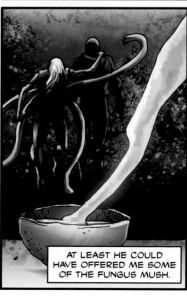

AT LEAST HE COULD HAVE OFFERED ME SOME OF THE FUNGUS MUSH.

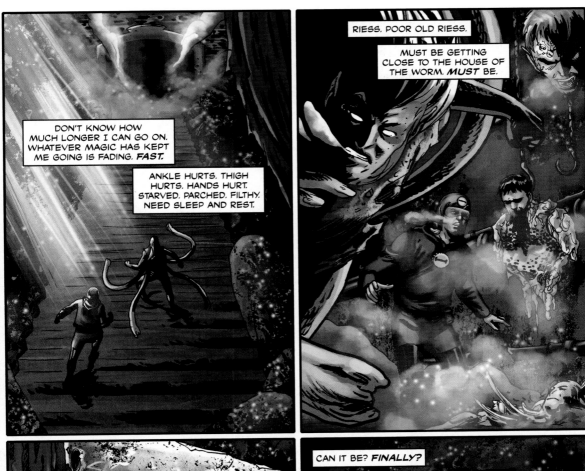

DON'T KNOW HOW MUCH LONGER I CAN GO ON. WHATEVER MAGIC HAS KEPT ME GOING IS FADING. *FAST.*

ANKLE HURTS. THIGH HURTS. HANDS HURT. STARVED. PARCHED. FILTHY. NEED SLEEP AND REST.

RIESS, POOR OLD RIESS.

MUST BE GETTING CLOSE TO THE HOUSE OF THE WORM. *MUST* BE.

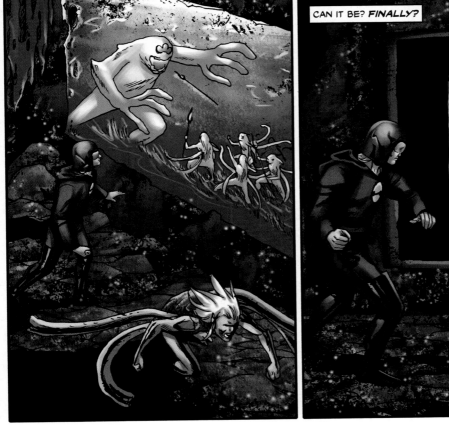

CAN IT BE? *FINALLY?*

THE WAY *HOME.*

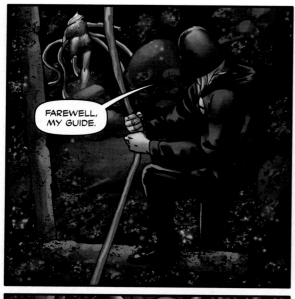

FAREWELL, MY GUIDE.

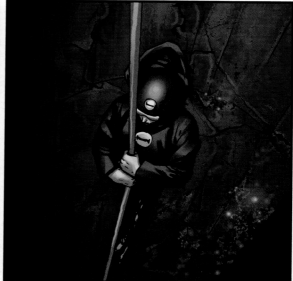

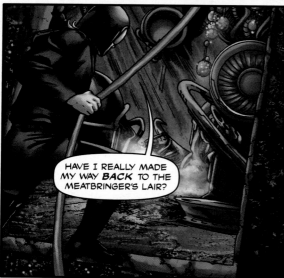

HAVE I REALLY MADE MY WAY *BACK* TO THE MEATBRINGER'S LAIR?

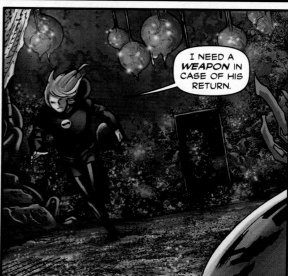

I NEED A *WEAPON* IN CASE OF HIS RETURN.

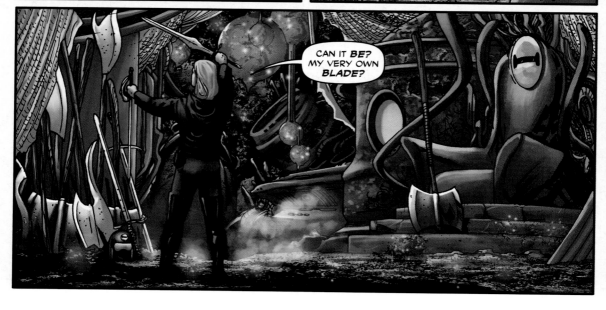

CAN IT *BE?* MY VERY OWN *BLADE?*

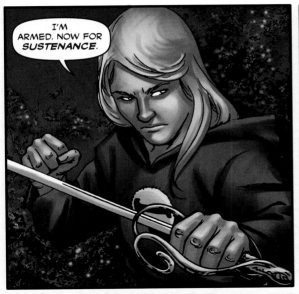

I'M ARMED. NOW FOR *SUSTENANCE*.

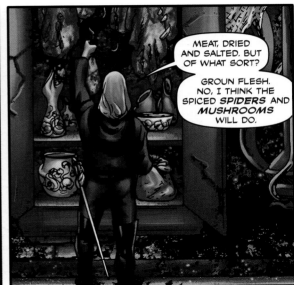

MEAT, DRIED AND SALTED. BUT OF WHAT SORT?

GROUN FLESH. NO, I THINK THE SPICED *SPIDERS* AND *MUSHROOMS* WILL DO.

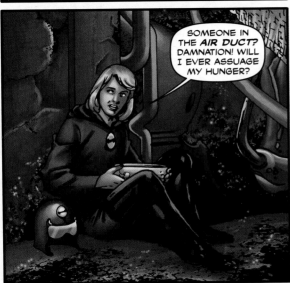

SOMEONE IN THE *AIR DUCT?* DAMNATION! WILL I EVER ASSUAGE MY HUNGER?

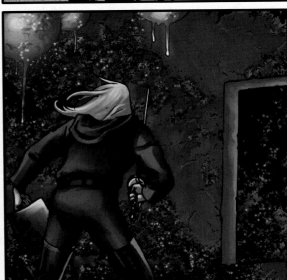

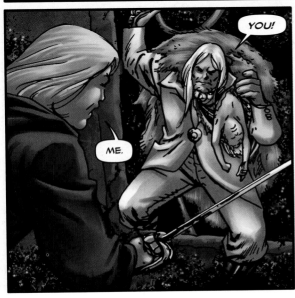

YOU!

ME.

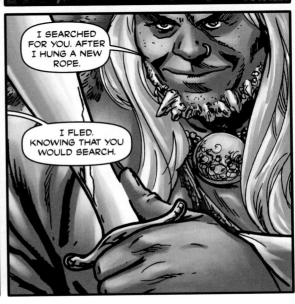

I SEARCHED FOR YOU. AFTER I HUNG A NEW ROPE.

I FLED. KNOWING THAT YOU WOULD SEARCH.

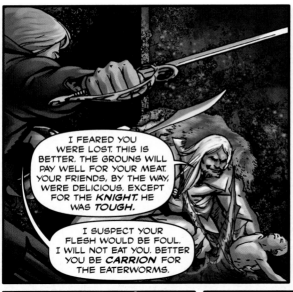

I FEARED YOU WERE LOST. THIS IS BETTER. THE GROUNS WILL PAY WELL FOR YOUR MEAT. YOUR FRIENDS, BY THE WAY, WERE DELICIOUS, EXCEPT FOR THE *KNIGHT.* HE WAS *TOUGH.*

I SUSPECT YOUR FLESH WOULD BE FOUL. I WILL NOT EAT YOU. BETTER YOU BE *CARRION* FOR THE EATERWORMS.

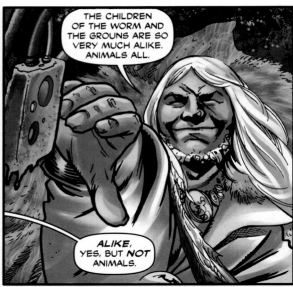

THE CHILDREN OF THE WORM AND THE GROUNS ARE SO VERY MUCH ALIKE. ANIMALS ALL.

ALIKE, YES, BUT *NOT* ANIMALS.

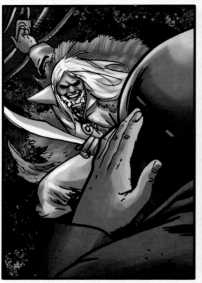

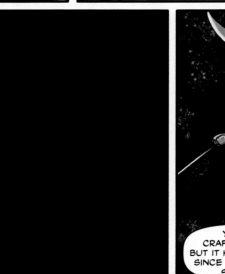

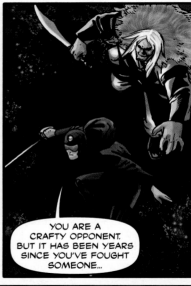

YOU ARE A CRAFTY OPPONENT. BUT IT HAS BEEN YEARS SINCE YOU'VE FOUGHT SOMEONE...

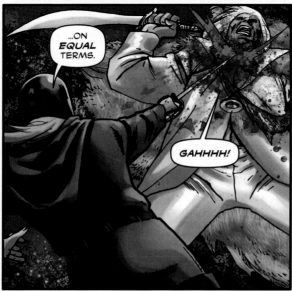

...ON *EQUAL* TERMS.

GAHHHH!

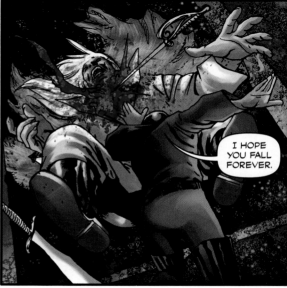

I HOPE YOU FALL FOREVER.

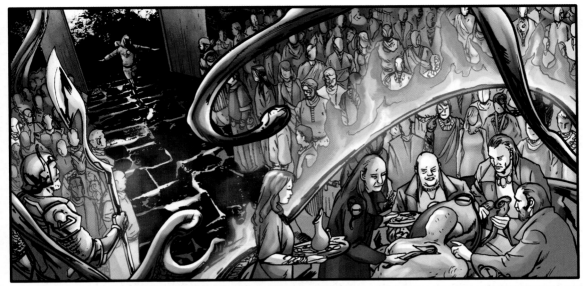

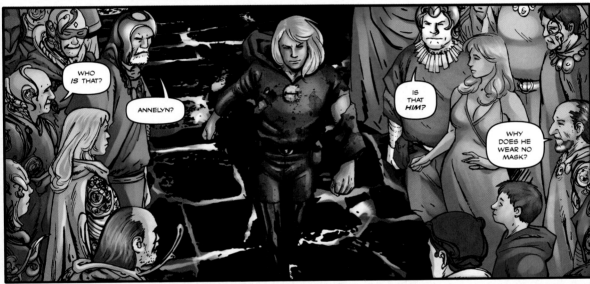

WHO *IS* THAT?

ANNELYN?

IS THAT *HIM*?

WHY DOES HE WEAR NO MASK?

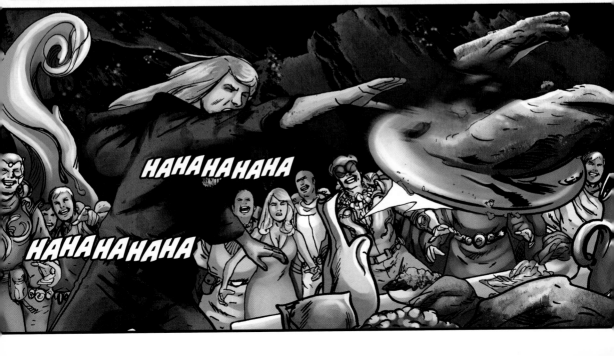

HAHAHAHAHA

HAHAHAHAHA

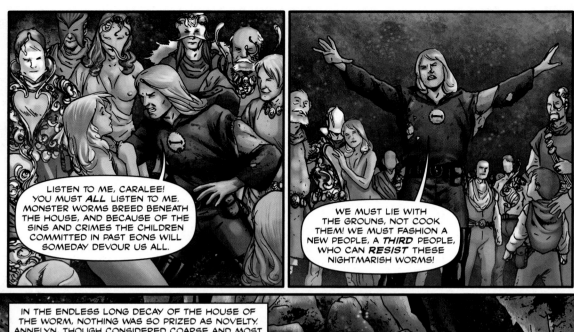

LISTEN TO ME, CARALEE!
YOU MUST *ALL* LISTEN TO ME.
MONSTER WORMS BREED BENEATH
THE HOUSE, AND BECAUSE OF THE
SINS AND CRIMES THE CHILDREN
COMMITTED IN PAST EONS WILL
SOMEDAY DEVOUR US ALL.

WE MUST LIE WITH
THE GROUNS, NOT COOK
THEM! WE MUST FASHION A
NEW PEOPLE, A *THIRD* PEOPLE,
WHO CAN *RESIST* THESE
NIGHTMARISH WORMS!

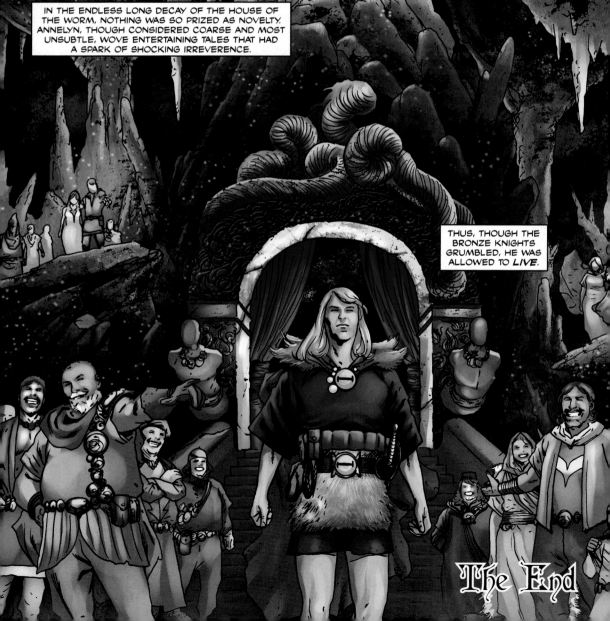

IN THE ENDLESS LONG DECAY OF THE HOUSE OF
THE WORM, NOTHING WAS SO PRIZED AS NOVELTY.
ANNELYN, THOUGH CONSIDERED COARSE AND MOST
UNSUBTLE, WOVE ENTERTAINING TALES THAT HAD
A SPARK OF SHOCKING IRREVERENCE.

THUS, THOUGH THE
BRONZE KNIGHTS
GRUMBLED, HE WAS
ALLOWED TO *LIVE*.

The End

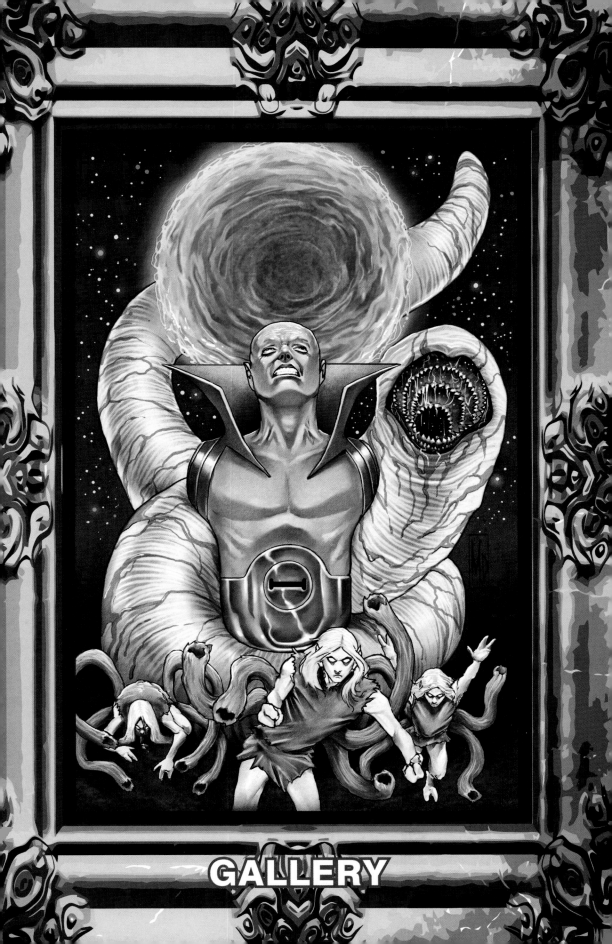

GALLERY

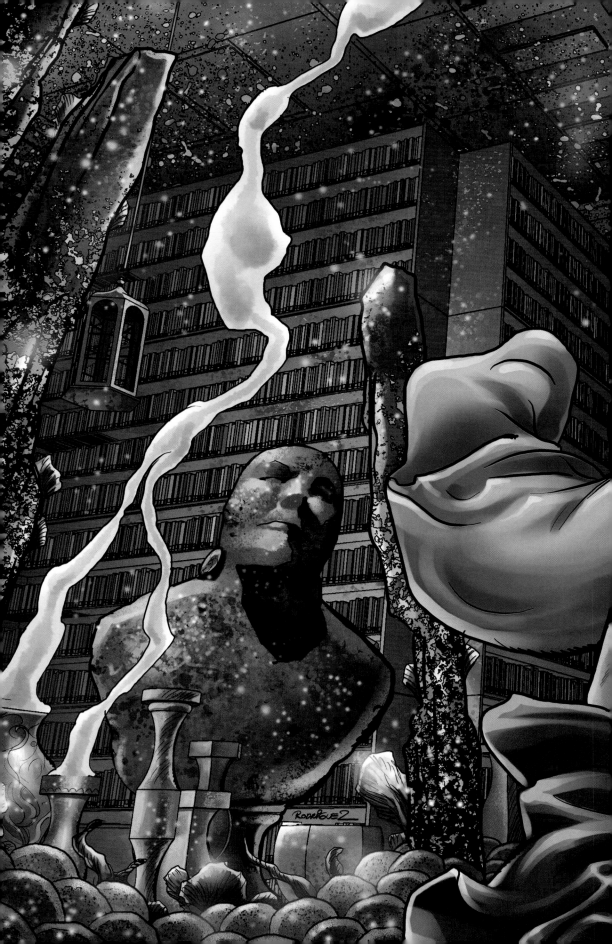

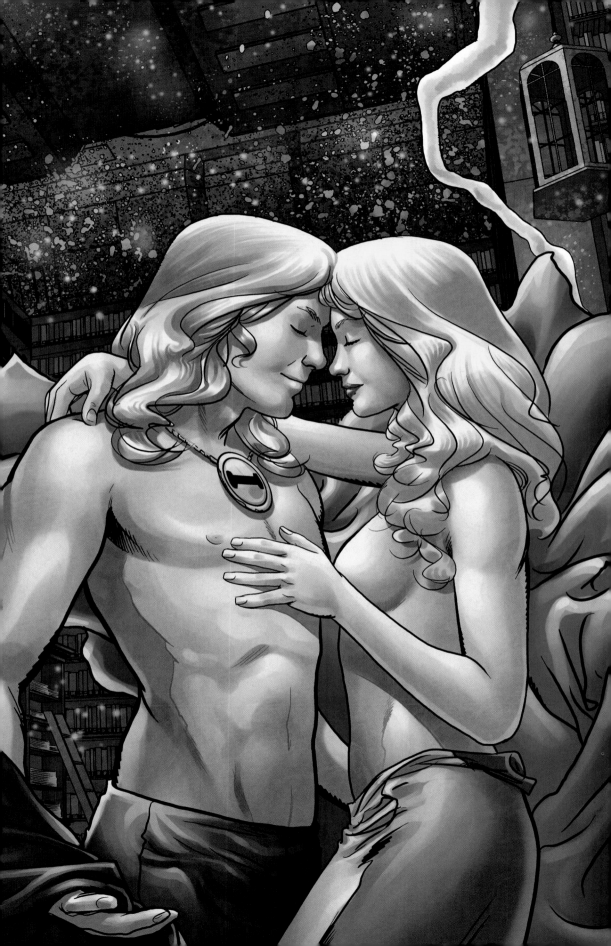

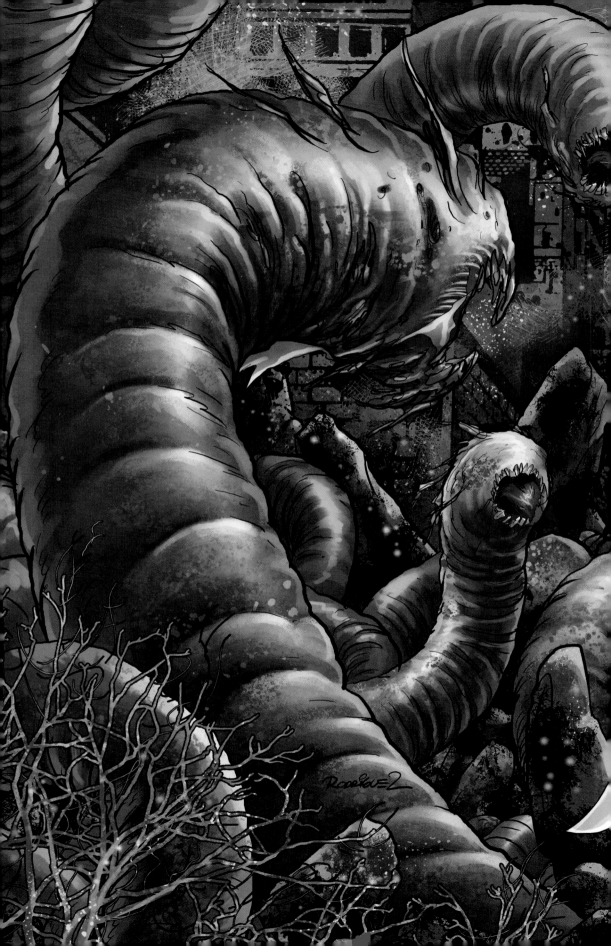

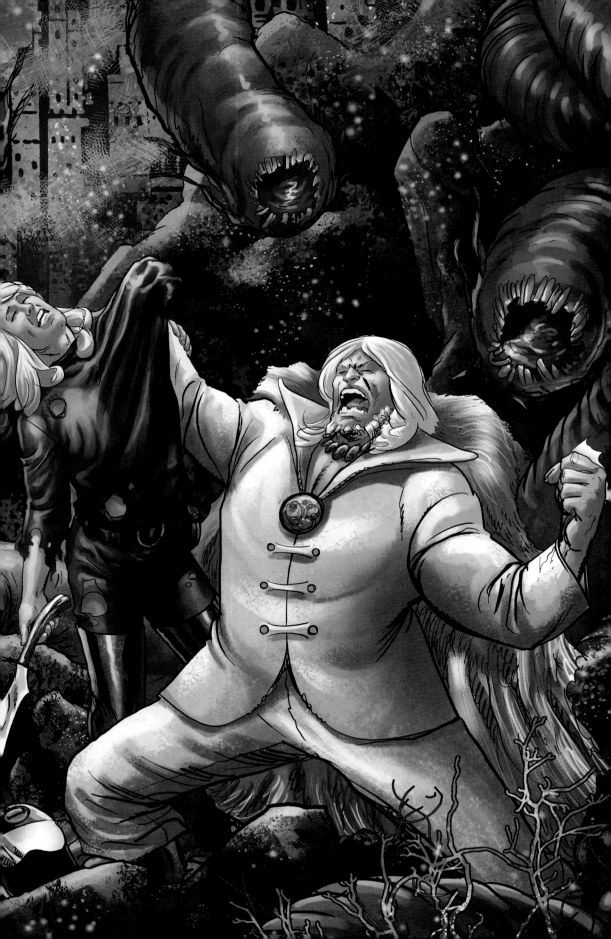

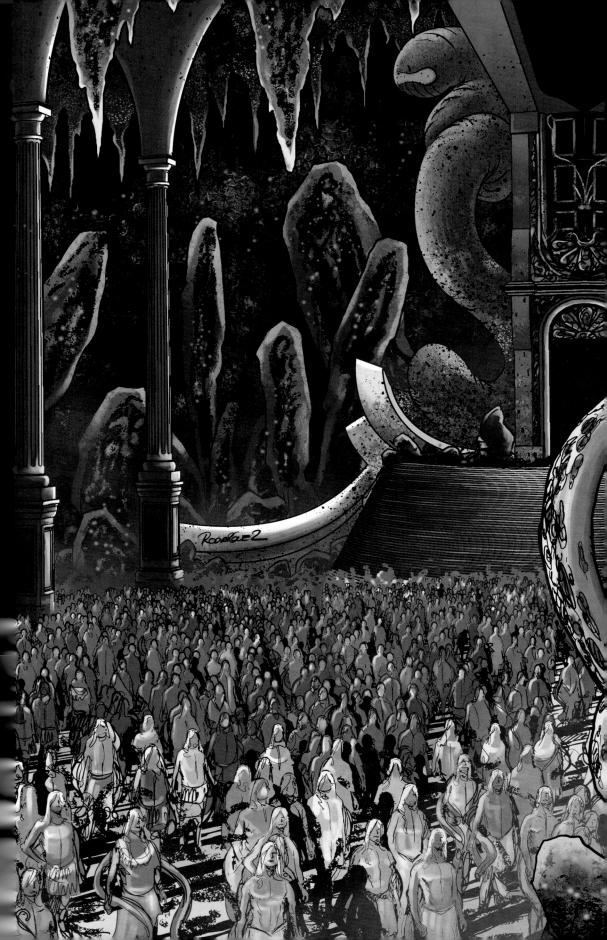

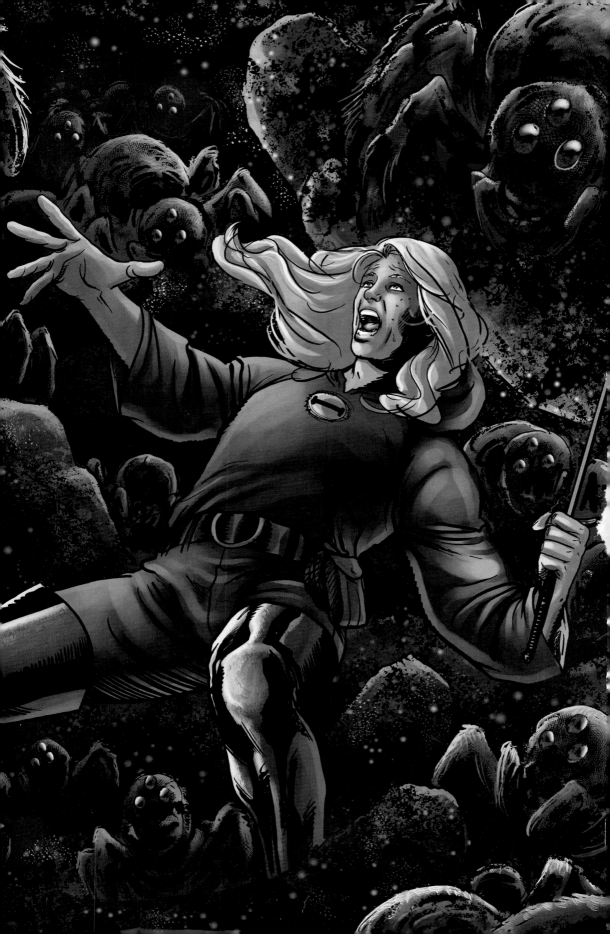

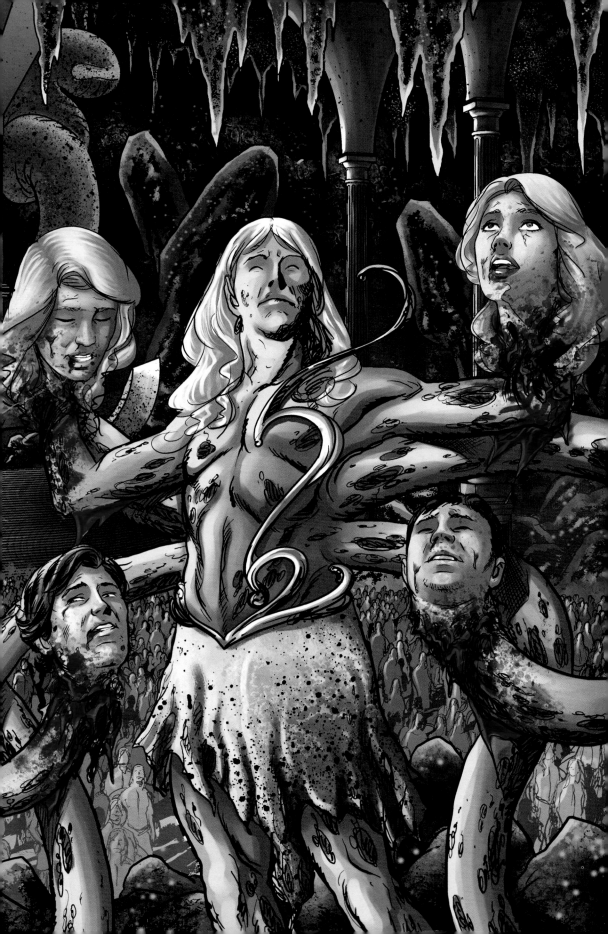